Conquering Stroke

Conquering Stroke

*How I Fought My Way Back
and How You Can Too*

Valerie Greene

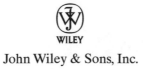

John Wiley & Sons, Inc.

Published by John Wiley & Sons, Inc., Hoboken, New Jersey
Published simultaneously in Canada

Photo credits: page 133, © Brion Price Photography; page 150, © Iman Photography; all other photos courtesy of the author

The information contained in this book is not intended to serve as a replacement for professional medical advice. Any use of the information in this book is at the reader's discretion. The author and the publisher specifically disclaim any and all liability arising directly or indirectly from the use or application of any information contained in this book. A health care professional should be consulted regarding your specific situation.

Limit of Liability/Disclaimer of Warranty: While the publisher and the author have used their best efforts in preparing this book, they make no representations or warranties with respect to the accuracy or completeness of the contents of this book and specifically disclaim any implied warranties of merchantability or fitness for a particular purpose. No warranty may be created or extended by sales representatives or written sales materials. The advice and strategies contained herein may not be suitable for your situation. You should consult with a professional where appropriate. Neither the publisher nor the author shall be liable for any loss of profit or any other commercial damages, including but not limited to special, incidental, consequential, or other damages.

For general information about our other products and services, please contact our Customer Care Department within the United States at (800) 762-2974, outside the United States at (317) 572-3993 or fax (317) 572-4002.

Wiley also publishes its books in a variety of electronic formats. Some content that appears in print may not be available in electronic books. For more information about Wiley products, visit our web site at www.wiley.com.

Library of Congress Cataloging-in-Publication Data

Greene, Valerie, date.
  Conquering stroke : how I fought my way back and how you can too / Valerie Greene.
    p. cm.
  Includes bibliographical references and index.
  ISBN 978-0-470-13792-5 (cloth)
 1. Greene, Valerie, 1964- —Health. 2. Cerebrovascular disease—Patients—United States—Biography. I. Title.
  RC388.5.G727 2008
  362.196'810092—dc22
  [B]
                                                     2008001365

Printed in the United States of America

10 9 8 7 6 5 4 3 2 1

In loving memory of my father,
who always believed in me.

Thanks, Dad,
your little "B" did it!

Contents

Foreword

In this time of transition from the classical methods for treating stroke patients to the new ones emphasizing prevention and emergency management to restore function, we are fortunate to have people such as Valerie Greene who, tragically, suffered a devastating stroke that could have ruined her life. With excellent treatment and "true grit" on her part, she overcame most of her horrible disability and now, all of us, both professionals and public alike, are learning what a stroke is like and what one can do to prevent and to recover from a stroke. This is essential because those of us who have not suffered one can only imagine how it ruins one's life!

Valerie has done it, and yes, she tells us her story as well as describes the cutting edge of prevention and therapy, using not only traditional but also alternative methods to put herself back in the mainstream of society and to restore her as a civic leader. She has written a gripping autobiography full of thought-provoking information and ideas for all of us to embrace.

I am proud to know her.

James F. Toole, M.D.
President of the International Stroke Society
The Walter C. Teagle Professor of Neurology
and Professor of Public Health Sciences
Wake Forest/Baptist Medical Center
Winston-Salem, North Carolina

Acknowledgments

Thank you, God, for restoring my body, mind, and spirit. I am so grateful! You have brought me such a long way safely through the fire. I am so grateful for all the angels and guides you sent to protect, encourage, and support me, especially my loving family and friends.

My deep appreciation to some powerful women who were a constant source of support to me, personally and in helping complete this book: Cindi Sholander, Nancy Johnson, Donna Harris, Vivienne Bailey, Markay Holly-Schroeder, Donna Eden, Christina Monterastelli, Donna Griffin, and Rhonna Bodin.

I am also grateful for my agent extraordinaire, Maura Teitelbaum; my editor, Christel Winkler; and for all those who were involved at my publisher, John Wiley & Sons.

Many thanks to Catherine Revland for her hard work, research, and commitment to this project, and for her faithful collaboration with a team of people who have brought this book to fruition.

My sincere gratitude to all the physicians who contributed their insight and expertise: Rhett Bergeron, M.D.; Svetlana A. Dambinova, D.Sc., Ph.D.; David J. Dickoff, M.D.; Richard O. Fass, M.D.; James L. Frey, M.D.; William S. Maxfield, M.D.;

Richard A. Neubauer, M.D.; James F. Toole, M.D.; Joseph D. Weissman, M.D.; Mojka Renaud, L.N., Dipl., A.C.N.C.C.A.; and Terese A. Uliano, M.A., C.C.C.-S.L.P.

And for my partner, Marlies, who has accompanied me on this journey and continues to travel the road ahead with me.

Introduction

—◆◆◆—

Twelve years ago, at age thirty-one, I was riding high. I had a successful career, a fancy car, a posh address, a closet full of designer-label clothes, and more friends than I could name. Then without any warning, it all fell apart when in June 1996 I suffered a catastrophic stroke. It was one of the worst kinds, caused by a large blood clot that blocked my basal artery, where all routes to the brain merge into one. You don't hear too much about this form of stroke, as nine out of ten victims die immediately. Although I was one of the lucky few, it left me half paralyzed, deaf in one ear, and unable to speak or even swallow. The doctors told me I would probably never walk again.

Like most patients in the aftermath of a massive stroke, I sank into a deep abyss. When three psychiatrists came into my room and tried to encourage me to accept my limitations, it felt like a death sentence. But instead of succumbing to it, something deep within me resisted. That moment ignited a spark that grew in strength during the weeks that followed, firing up my determination to begin the fight of my life. I just didn't know how to begin. My thinking was disoriented and I couldn't express myself verbally or in writing. I was trapped,

1

a prisoner within my own body, with no path of escape in sight.

Over time, I slowly regained my strength and clarity of thought. It was then that I began to educate myself, gathering information about every therapy that promised to restore me to health. My search turned into a twelve-year odyssey of recovery, a process of trial and error during which I tried every available treatment I could afford, discarded the ones that didn't work, and continued with the ones that did.

Today I am a walking, talking miracle. Whenever I speak before a group of stroke survivors, they respond with hope, applauding from their wheelchairs when they see me walking unassisted to a microphone. My presence alone reenergizes them because of the message I bring that recovery is possible, even from the most debilitating kind of stroke. I have written this book to share with every survivor and caregiver the valuable information I have learned during my recovery, some of it hard to come by, describing the procedures that worked for me and that may work for anyone searching for a way to heal from a stroke.

Although Western medicine is the best in the world when it comes to intervention, it has little to offer stroke victims after the crisis is over in the way of recovery. More and more people are investigating beyond conventional medicine when they want to get well, and my experience led me to do the same. The therapies in this book represent the full spectrum of global medicine—everything that works, not just what's profitable. Some of these regenerative therapies are a well-kept secret in the United States, even though they have long track records of effectiveness in other countries. I have given special emphasis to the little-known treatments that worked wonders for me. You will find a resource section after each chapter.

The most valuable treatment I want to share is the one medical science can't account for. I discovered it shortly after being released from the hospital while sitting on my front porch swing, overcome with fear and frustration and considering suicide. It changed me forever.

In my upscale neighborhood it is a major faux pas to sit on the front porch of your home, but I was so lonely and eager to connect with others that I put aside all social graces. Each day I would sit there and wait for the mailman, slowly rocking back and forth with my one good foot while my paralyzed left foot hung limp at the end of my lifeless left leg. As I rocked and waited, desperate thoughts would come to my mind. I was willing to do whatever it took to find a way out of this nightmare and to resuscitate my inert body. One morning, out of nowhere, an idea came to me: *When I can stop this swing with my left foot, I'll know there's hope.*

Day after day I sat on my porch and challenged that foot. I even invented a little game in which my right side became a cheerleader for my left side, encouraging it to move: *Come on, I really need you. I know you're terribly traumatized, but we've got to work together. You can do it. I know you can!* It sounds silly, but I was driven to continue, because it was all I knew that I could do for myself, and I had to do something. Days turned into weeks and my self-pep talks continued, urging my left side to wake up and get back in the game.

Though I was clueless at the time, I was actually doing something important. I was reactivating a neural pathway between my brain and my body. Then one day, long after I had given up any real hope that it would ever happen, my left foot stopped the swing. It moved! I've heard about rescue workers, digging for survivors after an earthquake, who hear faint cries below the rubble. They begin to dig with all their might, pulling off the layers of devastation, excited as they hear voices calling out "I'm here!" I felt that same excitement. Somewhere, imprisoned deep within my paralyzed body, I was alive, and I had found a way to dig myself out.

Of all the recovery therapies in this book, the most powerful was my spirit that drove my mind to move my left foot for the first time. Afterward, I could never be hopeless again. If I could use my mind to restore movement to my paralyzed left foot, I felt I could do anything. From that day forward I trained my mind with the same determination I began training my body— diligently, repeatedly, patiently, surmounting one obstacle and then another, feeling stronger each time. One day I framed my cane and hung it on my living room wall. It's still there, a trophy of my victory over this disease.

Early in my recovery, I promised that if I ever got my voice back, I would never stop sharing my story. I've kept my word. Not in my wildest dreams did I foresee the day when I would have the opportunity to become a voice for millions of stroke survivors, in a position to share how I went from a powerless, hopeless, tangled mess to a walking, talking miracle. I can speak for them because I know what they're going through. A stroke is an incredibly cruel and devastating disease, one of the few that can lay waste not only to the body and the mind but also the spirit. The loss of all three is unfathomable for anyone but another stroke survivor. As one person put it, "Having a stroke is like an earthquake to your mind, body, and spirit."

I, too, was once overpowered by grief and despair, unwilling to take the first step toward getting well. But I now know that it is possible for stroke survivors to break through that paralysis of mind, body, and spirit. I'm living proof that it can be done, even for those who have had a catastrophic stroke. The healing power of the human spirit is available to everyone. You may not realize it, but we can all have this fire within. It can propel you to accomplish great things, sometimes when you least expect them. The only way to find it is to take that first step toward trying.

The message I want to bring to every stroke survivor and caregiver is that there has never been more reason for hope. During the twelve years of my recovery, amazing progress has been made in all areas of stroke medicine. As a result, what was seen as a death sentence not so long ago is now a treatable, preventable disease. I have written this book to provide you with all the information you need about these new resources, and many more that are on the horizon, and to provide you with what is most important: hope. So let the journey begin!

1

The Day My Life Changed Forever

E VEN AS A CHILD I was a fighter. I can still imagine those six-shooters sliding down my then absent hips, the hem of my fringed skirt swishing across the back of my legs, and my bare toes squishing inside closed leather boots. I practiced my draw and got so good I could beat both my sisters. As the second of three daughters, I thought of myself as something like an Oreo cookie: the best part is the middle. They say the middle child is the peacemaker. Looking back, that sounds right. The chaos in our family demanded that someone could make peace.

But try as I might that June night in 1996, I could neither make peace nor find any. A war of my senses was raging in my head as I fought desperately to understand what was happening to my body and to make myself understood.

MONDAY, JUNE 10, 1996, 9:30 P.M.

What's happening to me? I can't focus, I can't keep my balance. "I-I-I-I-I nnnneeeed hhhhellllllp." I didn't recognize my own voice. My left side was weak and heavy, my speech was slurred, and I was tumbling through space.

5

What is wrong with me?

The view of my world had suddenly become a haze—distorted and nauseating. I felt as though I were stuck on Disney World's Mad Tea Party ride. My teacup would not stop spinning, this ride would not end.

The bright lights in the emergency room nearly blinded me as I lay in my curtained cubicle, trembling in fear. Across from my bed, a man—loud, obnoxious, and obviously drunk, was yelling obscenities. *Would anyone hear my genuine cries for help?*

"I-I-I-I neeeeeed helllp," I pleaded with the nurses. I was desperately trying to request that a nurse call a doctor who knew my history, but my words just ran together. Instead, I motioned for pen and paper and wrote my request, trying to steady my trembling hand.

"Call Dr. Powers," I wrote. Dr. Powers is a neurosurgeon and friend. He would know what to do. Fortunately, a nurse deciphered my plea and agreed to call him. Moments later she returned to tell me that he was out of the country attending a medical conference.

My heart sank as my mind raced frantically. *What's going to happen to me now?*

I grasped the metal guardrails of my hospital bed as the dizziness increased and everything spun out of control. I began to vomit down the side of the bed. My words became dim and weak as I begged for help. Through blurred vision I could see the nurses' station. Heads turned every so often, but no one seemed to notice me or hear my cries. *Why doesn't anyone seem concerned?*

I was cold and my body shook as my head lay pressed against the cold bars I clung to. Beads of moisture ran off my face, and the odor of vomit was appalling. My strength was waning as my warrior spirit rallied to fight. It felt like hours until an orderly noticed I had passed out lying in a pool of my own vomit. Rather than change the linens, he lifted my head and laid a towel over the soiled area and wiped off my face.

Looking up at him, my eyes pleaded in the absence of words, then scribbled the word "stroke." He explained that he was only helping out in the ER but would deliver the note to a nurse. As he disappeared from sight, I passed out.

"Honey, we are taking you down for a test," the nurse said. "It won't take long." Barely able to open my eyes, I was relieved that help had finally arrived. Someone must have received my note, and a CT scan had been ordered.

After the scan, I returned to my cubicle and rested, hoping I was finally going to be treated. But an hour passed and still no further word. Nor was there a sound coming from the drunken guy who shared my space. I suspected that he had either sobered up or had been given something to quiet him. Whatever the case, it was silent.

SHORTLY AFTER MIDNIGHT

My test results arrived. "Good news, honey: your test results have come back and they are normal. Nothing is wrong. You can go home."

What was intended to bring relief only served to alarm me all the more. Even in my weakened state, I knew I was headed for a showdown. I was facing the fight my life. I shook my head, vehemently, in disagreement and grabbed my pen and paper. There was no way that *nothing* was wrong.

"MRI! I need an MRI!" I scrawled. I knew that MRIs were more precise than CT scans.

"The MRI machine is down for repairs. Just get some rest, sweetie. I'm going to give you a shot that will help you sleep."

Rest? You want me to sleep? Are you crazy? Airlift me to another hospital! I've got to get an MRI! I'm having a stroke!

As I eyed the needle drawing closer, I realized that whatever she was injecting would mask my symptoms and silence my ability to advocate for my medical needs. All I could think was, *If I'm having a stroke, this is going to kill me.* You're *going to kill me.*

I was terrified. I knew that whatever had gripped me was lethal and that if I was sent home I would likely die alone. At least if I stayed here I would have people around me. My entire body quaked with fear. I threw my hands up, trying to demonstrate that this was simply not acceptable. *I can't leave! Something dreadful is happening to me!*

The nurse responded to my body language, "Honey, why would you want to stay here? Just go home and sleep it off."

I don't believe it! They think I'm drunk. Yet even in my fear and outrage, I could see it from their perspective. My youth, my slurred speech, and my stumbling had all contributed to a composite of a young woman who'd simply had one too many martinis.

No! As I reasoned further, I decided that it should be easy enough to determine an alcohol-induced stupor from a stroke. I refused to leave the hospital, insisting on more tests. I was then put on a waiting list for a room.

It's strange, but at thirty-one years of age, as a successful entrepreneur, fiercely independent, and stubbornly self-sufficient, I never imagined that, at the moment I would stare death in the eye, all I would want is my mother. Though she and I had had a strained relationship over the years, now she was all I wanted. I was breathless. The words spilled out, "Call my mother."

The large clock in the ER reminded me that it was after midnight, and I fretted at my mother's panic upon receiving this late-night call from the hospital. I wasn't sure she was home, or whether she was even in town. Fortunately she was. I was relieved. The nurse injected me with medication to relieve the nausea, and I fell asleep.

Two hours later I woke to my mother's gentle caress on my forehead, letting me know that she and my stepfather had arrived. I began to cry. In my broken state I tried desperately to explain, but words simply vanished as they reached my tongue.

"What's wrong with her?" Mother asked the nurse. "What's happened? Where's her doctor?" The nurse tried to explain that I had arrived earlier that evening, stumbling and with slurred speech.

"But what's causing her speech to be like that? Why can't she talk right?"

"We don't know," the nurse replied. "We suspect that something must have terribly frightened her to cause her to lose her voice."

I was horrified that the hospital personnel never considered that I might be having a stroke, especially since speech difficulty is a major symptom.

My mind raced anxiously, trying to figure out how I could prove that I was stroking. No one even seemed to be thinking in that direction. *But then, why would they? I was too young to be having a stroke.*

Yet, only a few months earlier, my neurosurgeon friend Dr. Powers had ordered an MRI because he suspected that the symptoms I had complained of over the previous six months could be stroke-related: sudden headache, extreme dizziness, slurred speech, and one-sided numbness. I felt sure that if they had access to copies of my earlier MRI it would prove that I could be having a stroke.

Once again I motioned for pen and paper, and my stepfather reached into his suit pocket and pulled out his pen. I began to write precise directions to the clinic where my MRI results could be found.

"Valerie," my stepfather said, "they're not going to be open right now, but I'll go as soon as they are." And he did.

Sometime in the early morning hours, I was finally moved to a room. I was physically and emotionally spent.

TUESDAY, JUNE 11, 10 A.M.

I awoke, surprised to be alive. More than twelve hours had passed, and still no neurologist had looked in on me. Two interns had read my chart and reassured my family and me that a neurologist had been called.

"All we can do is give her another injection to ease the nausea," they said to my mother. "We have her under observation."

My mother, the ever-consummate southern belle, always charming and respectful, politely replied, "Thank you. We appreciate your help."

Meanwhile, I'm dying and everybody's being nice! There I was, faint with frustration, my mutinous body ignoring my commands, my brain flickering on and off like a nearly burned-out bulb. Although the child in me urged "Valerie, you're tired; let go; we're done here," my spirit was all the while setting off fireworks. Guns blazing, my fiery will refused to quit. I was not going out without a fight.

The day passed as my strength continued to deteriorate. I vomited continuously until I finally passed out. By evening I was curled up in a fetal position, foaming at the mouth. I was losing all ability to speak or make any movements with my legs or arms.

I motioned that I wanted water. My mother asked the nurse, "Why can't she have water? She's so thirsty."

"Unfortunately," the nurse replied, "she can't have anything to drink until we determine if she's having a neurological event."

This was hard for both my mother and me to hear. As I lay there, I was flooded with memories of how Mom tenderly nursed me as I was growing up. Apple slices, carrot sticks, and celery. Homemade soup and vitamins. How it must have pained her to not even be able to offer her child a sip of water. I had had nothing to drink in more than twelve hours since arriving in the ER.

The door to my room slowly opened. In walked my mother's best friend, Edith. She was like an aunt to me. She took one look at me and blurted out, "Oh, dear God!" Reaching for my hand, she directed, "Valerie, squeeze my hand if you can hear me."

I squeezed as best I could.

"Frances," Edith ordered my mother, "get on your knees! We've got to pray!"

My mother and Edith knelt beside my hospital bed and prayed for God's help.

I sensed my life was fading. I was dying. My breathing slowed. The steady beeping of the heart monitor and the voices surrounding me faded into a velvety softness. The edges of the room became indistinct as my eyes closed. The nausea stopped, and I no longer felt pain. My body was shutting down. Still lying in a fetal position, my notepad clenched tightly in my hand, I scribbled these words: "Am I dying?"

My pain began to subside, and as the tension released, I suddenly felt no fear. I was safe and warm . . . enveloped . . . almost cocooned. As this tranquillity saturated my senses, I was engulfed by a brilliant white light. I knew of this light; I had heard it described, throughout my life, as the presence of God. Many medical personnel attribute this phenomenon to the neurological impact of the brain shutting down. Whatever the explanation, having experienced this firsthand, I can attest that its effect on me was to eliminate all fear of death.

As I gave myself over to this peace that is described as "passing all understanding," highlights of my life flashed before me like scenes from a movie on fast-forward, only slowing down to frame certain happy events. I saw myself at five years old, dressed in a fringed cowgirl miniskirt with a holster and guns; at seven years old, laughing with my sisters as we peeked out of our playhouse window; racing my father to the lake for our annual swim contest the summer I was sixteen; and crossing the finish line as I ran track in high school.

But I also saw less happy times. I saw myself looking for and not finding my father's shaving kit after my mother told us he had left; holding my beloved cat while she died; getting beaten up on my first day of public school in the sixth grade. While in the presence of the light, I felt no pain as I once again saw these hurtful events taking place. I simply felt an inexplicable, peaceful acceptance.

And then I saw a funeral. My mother and father weeping. My sisters sobbing. A multitude of friends gathered on the landscaped grounds of a cemetery. As I saw this scene, I slowly recognized that this was *my* funeral. I was watching my family weep for *me*. Their grief stirred something deep within and established a confidence within me that it was not my time to die. I shouted "No!" and suddenly I was jolted from that brilliant light, feeling as though I had broken the surface from beneath deep waters. I gasped for air.

Sometime during the night I lost consciousness and was moved to intensive care.

"Lie still!" a voice commanded as something sharp jabbed my right arm. A nurse was trying to insert an IV needle. She missed the vein, and it stung. I was not fully alert, and my instincts urged my left hand to cover the sting, but my left hand and my left arm would not cooperate. They were immobile. I was paralyzed!

Terrified, my brain reeled with a litany of questions. *What is wrong? Why can't I move my arm and leg? What is going on?* As I lost consciousness once again, I prayed, "*Dear God, please help me.*"

WEDNESDAY, JUNE 12, 10 A.M.

I woke to the sound of my sister, Angela, and a man arguing in the hallway. Thirty-six hours after he was first called, a neurologist, Dr. Gonzales, finally arrived. My sister insisted that I was having a stroke. Sounding exasperated, he countered emphatically, "There is no way this girl is having a stroke. She's too young!" But Angie wouldn't back down.

"How do you know it's not a stroke? How can you be sure? Given her history, you *have* to rule out the possibility of stroke."

"To rule out all possibility of stroke I would have to do an angiogram," Dr. Gonzales replied.

"Do it! Do it now," Angie urged.

As my gurney was rushed through the hallway, Angie ran alongside, holding my hand, accompanied by my dear friend Andy, who was on the other side. As we paused at the door of the surgical area Angie whispered in my ear, "I love you. I'll see you soon." As the double doors swung shut, I heard her sobbing.

The room looked like an auto repair shop, with different-size tubes and hoses hanging from the wall. As I was placed on a cold metal table, a man wearing what looked like a welder's helmet with a glass shield covering his face told me that a small catheter would be inserted into my groin. A fluid would then be injected that would show if there were any blockages in my arteries. He explained the very real risk that if the needle punctured my artery wall I could die during the procedure.

I managed to scribble my signature, allowing them to proceed. Because of my condition, I could not be placed under anesthesia for fear I would not come out of it. An injection of local anesthesia numbed my leg. I watched on the monitor as a small tube was inserted into my right thigh and the dye was slowly injected. The dye showed up on the monitor as a white line traveling slowly up through my artery.

Hours later I opened my eyes, feeling Angie's hand holding mine, telling me to hold on and fight. I was in the critical care unit, lying in the bed, covered with sheets, my right leg bandaged to protect the wound made by the incision.

As the local wore off, my leg felt like it was burning, pain radiating upward. My sister handed me a cup of water, but I was too weak to hold it to my lips. Angie's hands shook with fear. When Dr. Gonzales came into the room to give the results of the test, the look on his face said it all. Something was terribly wrong. He explained the result of the angiogram to my family and drew a diagram to show what had happened.

The results were conclusive: I had suffered a massive brain stem stroke. A large blood clot had occluded the most vital artery leading to the brain. As a result my entire left side was paralyzed, leaving me unable to walk or talk. The message he delivered was surreal. Here I was, in the prime years of my life. I had known something was wrong, but this was too much for me to absorb—paralyzed, unable to speak, with most of my hearing lost.

"Miss Greene," Dr. Gonzales said, "the area in which this clot is positioned is inoperable. Therefore, we have started you on a heparin drip to dissolve the clot. However, I must inform you that if this is unsuccessful, the occlusion will stop the blood flow and end your life."

Whether I lived or died, there was no good news. If I left the hospital alive, I had to face the possibility of never walking or talking again. As the doctor delivered the prognosis, I could only watch his lips move. The news was just too horrifying to take in.

THURSDAY, JUNE 13

The aftermath of a stroke is much like the calm after a storm, but the peace is only an illusion. I lay in the critical care unit, barely alive, my body spent as I drifted into and out of sleep.

"Is there anything you would like?" Angie asked me. Exhausted and filled with despair, all I wanted was to be comforted. Waves of hunger washed over me, as did a fond memory of being out late at night with friends and stopping off at Krystal for those tiny burgers. I scribbled out my request: "Krystal."

Unsure at first, Angie soon figured out what I wanted. She knew, but I didn't realize that I was not allowed to have food. Still, she hurried to get what she thought might be my last request.

"Val, wake up." Someone was whispering my name. It was Angie. As I groggily opened my eyes I felt something pressed to my lips. *What is that smell? A Krystal burger? Why on earth would she bring me a Krystal burger?* She had torn the small

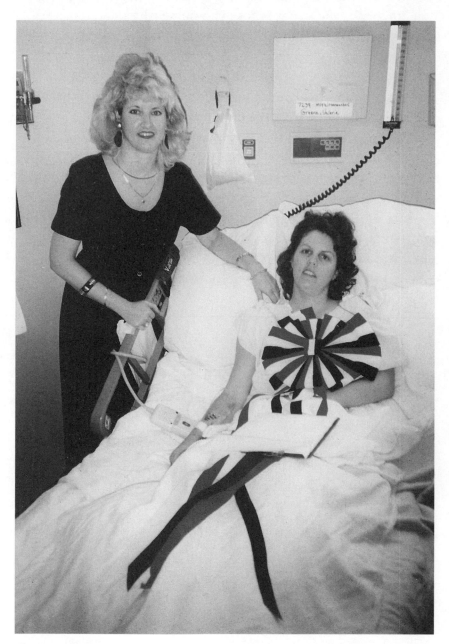

Angie and me

burger into tiny bites and like a mother feeding her young, she tried to entice me to eat before the nurses discovered us. Not remembering I had made the request, I turned my head away.

"Be strong, Val," Angie pleaded. "Please hold on. Remember when we were kids and we played cowgirls and Indians? You were always the leader, Val. You were so brave. Don't give up now. We all need you."

I felt something cold being placed into my right hand. It was a metal cap gun.

"Come on, Val," she said. "Remember how you never gave up without a good fight? Fight this. Be strong. You can do it."

I tried to grasp the gun, but it weighed as much as a bowling ball. Weakly I pressed it back into Angie's hand, willing her to understand that I couldn't be strong now. I couldn't fight. I needed somebody to be strong for me.

Vital Information

Now we have a drug we can call "Stroke Away."

—James L. Frey, M.D., director of the Stroke Program
at Barrow Neurological Institute of St. Joseph's
Hospital in Phoenix, Arizona; member of the Stroke
Advisory Board of the American Heart Association
and the American Stroke Association

IN JUNE 1996, the same month I had my stroke, the Food and Drug Administration approved a drug called tPA (Tissue Plasminogen Activator), which has transformed the way the medical profession perceives stroke—from a hopeless condition to a treatable disease. Patients treated with tPA have a 50 percent chance of having an excellent outcome, which constitutes a 30 percent better chance than without treatment. Because tPA must be given within three hours after the onset of a stroke, which is called the three-hour window, the American Heart Association and the American Stroke Association have established updated practice "Guidelines" that call for a new kind of response to stroke treatment. Not everyone who comes into the emergency department with stroke symptoms meets the requirements for receiving tPA, but *all* stroke patients benefit even indirectly from this new sense of urgency in stroke intervention.

Today, most metropolitan areas have fully equipped stroke centers where all personnel—EMS, nurses, CT scan techs, respiratory and lab personnel, emergency and neurological physicians—work together to meet time restrictions in transporting, diagnosing, and treating. Had I been given this kind of attention, there's a good chance that the massive stroke I suffered—and the twelve years I spent recovering—could have been prevented.

This is good news for people who live in or near a metropolitan area, but how about the ones who don't? Rarely is a hospital in a small town or a rural area equipped to provide the kind of optimum care that meets the new guidelines. Many of them don't even have a neurologist on staff, which leaves the emergency physicians without support in a life-or-death situation. Emergency physicians also may lack experience in examining neurological patients and evaluating CT scans. They have come under pressure to treat stroke patients with tPA, but they are fearful of using it without the guidance and involvement of neurologists.

James L. Frey, M.D., is director of the Stroke Program at Barrow Neurological Institute of St. Joseph's Hospital in Phoenix, Arizona, the fifth-largest metropolitan area in the country. After the introduction of tPA in 1996, Dr. Frey became aware of the problems faced by these emergency department doctors in outlying areas. "Emergency physicians have the responsibility for the outcomes of their patients, but they are uncomfortable with the sense of liability that comes with the FDA's approval of tPA, which requires emergency neurological evaluation, rapid explanation of benefits and risks, close, expert monitoring, and a 6 percent risk of serious brain hemorrhage. Emergency doctors were the guys on the front line, but they didn't have the neurological support they needed, so they tended to avoid using tPA to protect themselves from being sued in the event of a bad outcome. It didn't help that some of their thought leaders were poisoning the waters by misrepresenting the data about the drug in medical journals and other publications, sometimes scandalously. It was really a very difficult situation."

Determined to find a way to provide support for these reluctant emergency physicians, Dr. Frey instituted an outreach program at Barrow to meet their needs. He was fortunate to have the cooperation of Native American Air, a regional paramedic air ambulance company, which offered to fly him to outlying hospitals for free. There he discovered that the local paramedics and emergency physicians proved to be uniformly eager to participate in the use of tPA, once they knew they had the support of neurologists who would consult with them emergently and accept the patients in transfer.

At each venue, local paramedics and emergency room medical staff were given training in protocols for rapid response and treatment. Subsequently, when patients with stroke arrived at their hospitals, the emergency physicians received neurological support by telephone from the stroke team at Barrow, helping them determine the patient's eligibility for receiving tPA and administering it before air transportation to the stroke center for follow-up care. This method was nicknamed "drip and ship."

Previously, stroke centers dealt with telephone calls from other emergency departments with a "ship and drip" approach—the calling hospital would have to transport the stroke victim to the stroke center for tPA. That method lost precious time and has now been supplanted with more liberal telephonic support in many areas of the country.

Other stroke centers had used a "trip and treat" approach, in which stroke specialists would drive to the local hospitals and assist in giving the tPA prior to transport. That method proved to be too labor-intensive, however.

The drip and ship method at Barrow proved to be so successful that the program expanded to forty-three outlying hospitals from as far as 277 miles away, with an average flight time to the stroke center of thirty minutes.

In 2005, Dr. Frey and his team published "tPA by telephone: extending the benefits of a comprehensive stroke center," a study that reviewed their experience by comparing patient outcomes between those treated by telephone and those treated during the same time in the emergency department at Barrow. The results are pretty astonishing: the outreach program had increased the use of tPA by 72 percent in just two and a half years.

Since then, the stroke program at Barrow Neurological Institute has reviewed its ten-year experience with more than four hundred patients treated with tPA and found that implementation of a coordinated stroke team effort focusing on rapid processing of patients within its emergency department, together with those helped by telephone, has more than *tripled* the number of stroke patients who receive tPA—from 8 percent to up to 30 percent. The team also saw no more adverse events in their patients than were seen in *either* the original Barrow publication *or* in the National Institute of Neurological Disorders and Stroke (NINDS) publication that led to the approval of tPA for stroke in the *New England Journal of Medicine* (1995; 333: 1581–7).

"This is very suggestive evidence that expensive technology like telemedicine may not be necessary to improve patient care in an outreach program," Dr. Frey concludes. "You can do it with a cell phone. That's the most worthy objective to emphasize— we have something that works, and I know that the other institutions that have adopted telephonic support systems have experienced similarly gratifying results. There is now a lot of appropriate pressure on stroke centers to extend themselves by helping other hospitals that have fewer resources. If you're a concerned physician who wants the best for stroke patients, there's very little excuse for not doing this."

Dr. Frey also describes a movement that is under way to study telemedicine for stroke. Telemedicine involves the use of portable equipment that provides real-time audio and video communication between the treating emergency department and the stroke consultant: "The emergency department uses the portable device in the patient's room, where it can be moved about on wheels; 'zoom' in for close scrutiny during intricate examination of pupils, eye movements, facial asymmetry, and so forth; and allow direct verbal communication between the patient, the emergency department staff, and the consulting stroke neurologist. Control of the device is either in the hands of the consultant via his or her computer or in the hands of the emergency staff, in accordance with instructions from the consultant." Telemedicine equipment is costly, however, and further careful study of its utility is required before it can become a widespread approach to acute stroke care.

Hospitals with Stroke Centers

If you're reading this book, it's likely that you or a loved one is at high risk for this disease, or you have already experienced the major wake-up call that is a first stroke. These events can be seen as a terrifying crisis or a blessing, because they give people time to prepare for and even prevent the eventuality of a catastrophic brain attack. No longer are victims and their families helpless onlookers in the drama of the onset of a stroke. We now have a crucial role to play in the best possible outcome. I can't think of a more important goal to accomplish, or a greater reward.

In the resources section of this book you will find a list of stroke centers around the country, given state by state so you can locate the center nearest you. It is by no means complete because no official list exists right now, but by combining the "Get with the Guidelines" participant list of the American Heart Association and the American Stroke Association, the "Rapid Response" list of the National Stroke Association, the list of primary stroke centers certified by the Joint Commission for Accreditation of Healthcare Organizations, plus information on the Web sites of a number of state departments of health, the list in the back of this book is the most complete resource available at this time. Here is what a stroke center offers:

- Trained EMS workers

- Stroke teams, including a neurologist, on twenty-four-hour call
- Emergency room staff trained to follow the newest protocol
- Rapid diagnosis—no one put "under observation"
- State-of-the-art equipment and treatments, including promising new trials

Your nearest stroke center may be part of an outreach network to community hospitals. The best way to find out is to call your local hospital, because hometown EMS workers are most likely to be the ones who transport patients to the stroke center.

Am I Having a Stroke?

When people are having a heart attack, they may clasp their chest and say, "Call an ambulance!" But if their arm suddenly goes limp at their side, they might continue to watch TV and wait for the arm to get better. I know of a brain surgeon who ignored her symptoms and took a nap. She woke having a massive stroke. When it comes to a brain attack, it's not just knowledge that's important, it's also perception. An intact brain can perceive a damaged heart, but a damaged brain may not be able to perceive a damaged brain.

Unfortunately, the onset of a brain attack is not as obvious as the onset of a heart attack. Stroke symptoms may not be so dramatic, recognizable, or even painful, and they also vary, depending on what part of the brain is attacked. But the one thing the symptoms of a stroke have in common is that they happen suddenly—they *strike*.

About 80 percent of all strokes are ischemic (is-*kee*-mick), caused by a blood clot in an artery that blocks the delivery of oxygen to a part of the brain. The rest are hemorrhagic, caused by the leaking of blood into the brain through a burst blood vessel. Most major ischemic attacks are preceded by a transient ischemic attack (TIA) or ministroke. For this reason, even though these symptoms may be mild and don't last, they are still an emergency. Following are common symptoms of a TIA.

- A fleeting loss of vision in one or both eyes, like a shade being pulled down. Because the eye is the most sensitive detector of a sudden loss of blood flow, this symptom is a commonly recognized sign of a TIA.
- Sudden dizziness, trouble walking, or loss of coordination
- Sudden severe or unusual headache
- Loss of consciousness
- Sudden numbness, weakness, or tingling of the face or a limb, especially on one side of the body
- Sudden confusion or trouble speaking or understanding
- Difficulty in swallowing
- Any kind of function of the brain that is interrupted for a while—from a few minutes to up to twenty-four hours—and then returns

Seeking medical attention while you are having any of these symptoms is important. It allows physicians to evaluate whether you are having a stroke and to treat it. People who have had TIAs are at high risk for having a full stroke. Preventing that from happening may involve medication for treating high cholesterol or blood pressure, or it may be as simple as aspirin therapy.

The most commonly reported symptoms of an ongoing stroke are similar to those for a TIA, except that they don't go away.

Symptoms of a hemorrhagic stroke, caused by bleeding, can be the same as for an ischemic attack, but also can include the following:

- A sudden, intense headache at the outset that patients describe as a "thunderclap" or a "popping sound"
- A very large pupil that does not react to light
- Seizures

TAKE CHARGE!

If a computer loses power while recording a document, it can wipe out everything written since the last "save." The brain operates like that, too. It's why people often ask after they are interrupted, "Now, what was I saying?" When people are having a stroke, they also can be unaware of what just happened, but they are so incapacitated that they may deny it. If you see anyone who is showing signs of a stroke, step up to the plate. The following are three simple questions that can be highly accurate in determining whether a stroke is taking place:

1. Can they raise both arms above their head and keep them there?

2. Can they smile?

3. Can they speak a simple sentence without garbling words or slurring?

If a person has trouble responding to any of these questions, do not hesitate. Call an ambulance.

Strokes that attack the left hemisphere of the brain are more easily recognized because they affect speech, but when the right hemisphere is involved, symptoms may be more difficult to recognize or describe. In medical terms, they are called "awareness deficits."

The biggest problem in identifying stroke is that symptoms are so varied and subtle. Following is a list of what are called nontraditional symptoms.

- Pain in the face, chest, or limbs
- Disorientation
- Vomiting or flulike symptoms

- Inability to focus, such as loss of linear thought
- Shortness of breath
- An abrupt change in consciousness, described as a feeling of detachment from reality, or "being in la-la land"

Remember that you may not be aware of these symptoms because your brain has lost the ability to observe itself. This is why onlookers are so important when it comes to recognizing the symptoms of a stroke.

Why You Need to Dial 911

Time lost is brain lost, as the saying goes. Studies show that patients rushed to the hospital by ambulance are *seven times* more likely to receive tPA care than patients transported in other ways.

- Paramedics are trained to know the nearest fully equipped hospital and the fastest way to get there.
- The paramedics alert the emergency room that a possible stroke patient is arriving.
- The paramedics administer time-saving preliminary tests en route such as drawing blood, getting an IV line going, and conducting a preliminary neurological exam.
- Patients coming by ambulance are put on the "fast track" in the emergency room.

A caution: not every EMS team has been trained in the newest protocol, and you may be shocked to know that 911 medical dispatchers may not know much about stroke at all! One study of emergency response found that as many as one out of three dispatchers couldn't recognize the most common symptoms of a stroke, and when callers clearly said that a stroke was occurring, more than 50 percent of the dispatchers in the study did not code the call correctly. Nevertheless, in spite of the lack of knowledge that prevails about stroke, going by ambulance is still the best way to get treated, but you may need to be proactive. Here are some suggestions.

- Calls to 911 are always tape-recorded. If you don't think you're getting through to the dispatcher that you're having a stroke, don't hesitate to say in an authoritative voice, "Are you coding this call as a stroke? I must be taken by ambulance to ——— [the nearest comprehensive stroke center by name]."

- In some states (Massachusetts is one), EMS workers are required by law to bypass hospitals that are not certified by the state to admit stroke patients.

- If your state doesn't have such a mandate, know that people have the right to be taken to the hospital of their choice, as long as it's a reasonable distance away. Even though it may take more time to get there, it's far better than going to a hospital where they aren't prepared to treat you for stroke at all! If you get resistance from the ambulance team, don't hesitate to bring up the subject of liability.

Ruling Out a Bleed

Once patients arrive in the emergency room, many things must happen quickly. After a preliminary workup and medical history, diagnosis begins. This diagnosis is crucial, because treating a hemorrhagic stroke with a blood thinner, or an ischemic attack with an anticoagulant, can be fatal in both cases.

Following are procedures commonly used to diagnose a stroke:

- Computed tomography (CT or CAT) scan of the head and face is the first diagnostic test given to someone who comes into an emergency room with stroke symptoms, because it quickly shows whether a stroke is hemorrhagic or ischemic. It uses low-dose X-rays to take cross-section photos of the brain that will detect bleeding in or around the brain. Although it can rule out a bleed, it cannot detect the presence of damaged brain tissue that indicates an ischemic stroke. This is why it is so important to have a neurologist available in those crucial hours after a stroke, as he or she is trained to recognize the symptoms of an ischemic stroke and how to treat it.

- Magnetic resonance imaging (MRI) takes precise images of lesions, areas of dead brain cells caused by an ongoing or prior stroke, that show where tissue damage has taken place and the extent of the damage. The test is given in a special room, free of metal, as it involves a powerful magnetic field. Its drawback is the time it takes to get results—an hour, or a third of the three-hour window lost waiting for a diagnosis. It also can't be given to anyone with medical devices or other metallic objects that can't be removed. For this reason an MRI is not the diagnostic scan of choice. A CT scan does not always provide a clear diagnosis, however, in which case an MRI may be necessary before treatment can begin.

Treatment of an Ischemic Stroke

Standard treatment of a blockage has been the use of anticoagulants, such as heparin or warfarin, or other methods of thinning the blood. In some circumstances, surgery may be required to restore circulation. Following is an explanation of the new treatments.

- Tissue plasminogen activator (tPA), also known as a clot-buster, dissolves the clot. It must be given within three hours after onset because, after that time, blood vessel walls lose their viability (much like a leaky pipe will flood the surrounding area), causing blood to escape into the brain.

- MERCI retriever, short for mechanical embolus retrieval in cerebral ischemia, is another new procedure that removes the clot instead of dissolving it. A tiny instrument shaped like a corkscrew is inserted in an artery in the groin, and the clot is removed through a catheter. Because blood thinning does not take place, this procedure can extend the three-hour window of treatment to as many as eight hours.

To receive tPA, patients must first be given blood tests, pressure readings, and a CT scan that rules out a hemorrhagic stroke. If the results of these preliminary tests meet the necessary requirements, patients must also:

- know the time of onset of symptoms;
- not have had a stroke or a TIA within the past three months;
- not have had a seizure at the onset;
- not have had surgery within the past two weeks;
- not have been pregnant or nursing within the past month.

Treatment of a Hemorrhagic Stroke

This is the deadliest form of a stroke, responsible for 30 percent of all stroke deaths. Patients with this kind of stroke are often deeply sedated to help stop the flow of blood. The former Israeli prime minister Ariel Sharon suffered this kind of stroke, and he has been in a medically induced coma since January 2006.

As most hemorrhagic stroke patients have hypertension, reducing blood pressure levels is also a common procedure. Coagulants are given for the same reason. If a blood clot is involved in the rupture of the vessel and is in an area where it can be removed, surgery may be advocated. In other cases, blood may be drained from the brain to reduce pressure on the surrounding tissues.

Researchers are working around the world to find more effective ways to treat hemorrhagic stroke, and some promising new treatments are now in clinical trial.

- Recombinant Factor VII is a drug that has been approved for treating patients with hemophilia. It is now being studied by a neurologist at Columbia University for treatment of brain hemorrhages.

- Neurosurgeons in England are conducting trials to determine whether the most effective treatment is medications or surgery.

- A neurologist at the Johns Hopkins Hospital is conducting two clinical trials to determine whether small doses of tPA can be used to treat hemorrhagic stroke.

The past decade has seen an incredibly rapid change in stroke medicine, so much so that it's being called "the decade of the brain," "a revolution," and "a paradigm shift in thinking." David Dickoff, M.D., is chief of neurology at St. John's Riverside Hospital in Yonkers, New York, where he helped establish the stoke unit. His comments reflect those of many physicians who have been on the front lines during this time: "We are at the beginning of a beautiful journey in stroke medicine. Before the advent of tPA there had always been a sense of therapeutic nihilism regarding the treatment of stroke. There was no way to restore blood circulation; no way to remove a clot; and doctors, patients, and families were forced to take a wait-and-see attitude. Now there is absolutely no excuse to have that approach."

The public can be part of that journey by keeping up with the avalanche of information made public every day. By interviewing the top researchers in the field, I've done the best I can to include the most up-to-date information in this book— but there will be more available tomorrow. Fortunately, we now have the Internet, an excellent way of remaining informed without having to leave home. In the resources section at the back of this book you will find a number of reliable Web sites where you can get the latest breakthrough news in stroke medicine.

If You've Already Had a Stroke

Advanced treatments are already expanding the three-hour window, with more in the pipeline or in clinical trial, but the most important factor in successful stroke treatment and prevention is still an educated survivor. Here's what you can do right now.

- Research the nearest comprehensive stroke center by using the information provided in the resources section at the back of this book.

- If you haven't seen a neurologist or a stroke specialist and gotten a full workup, do so. Don't hesitate to get a second opinion.

- Keep your medical records and test results readily available, including the names of medications you are taking and their dosage. Better yet, maintain this information online or scan it on a memory stick.

- Call—or have someone else call—911 at the first sign of symptoms and make sure the dispatcher acknowledges that you're having a stroke.

- Alert your neurologist, but don't delay getting to the hospital waiting for a callback!

- If possible, take someone with you to the hospital to be your advocate, or call someone who knows your medical history to meet you there.

- At the hospital, be ready to report the time of onset, if possible, and to describe symptoms accurately and in detail.

- Find out the reasons for any delay—in those crucial hours following onset there shouldn't be any! And don't be afraid to be assertive. It may make all the difference.

Too many good brains have already been lost to a stroke. Now—through medical progress, patient education, and speed—others can be saved.

2

Early Warning

ORLANDO, FLORIDA, in the mid 1990s was very much as it is today, with a vibrant economy and a population steadily trending younger. I made my home in Winter Park, drove a nice car, and was quickly checking off each of my life goals on my "to do" list. I ran a thriving business, worked hard, and took good care of myself. I didn't smoke. My blood pressure was normal. I wasn't overweight or diabetic. So how did a young, healthy, highly motivated, entrepreneurial person like myself end up in a hospital bed, half paralyzed by a massive stroke?

I've learned since then that there's another risk factor—stress—that is rarely listed as a warning sign for stroke. Why a person's emotional state is ignored as a risk factor for this disease is unimaginable to me, yet it is, and I've made it my mission to tell people the role stress played in the months leading up to my stroke.

Stress is like the perfect storm. When conditions are just right, it can kill or disable you.

Before my stroke, I was a type A overachiever. Every morning I would rise before dawn and begin my day with a rigorous workout at the gym. At the office by eight in the morning, I would have a power lunch at noon, keep appointments all afternoon, and network at night. I wanted to be a millionaire before I was thirty.

Even as a child, if someone advised me it couldn't be done, I'd find a way to do it. I learned persistence from my dad. Success was in my genes because of him. His office wall was covered with awards for his business acumen. Dad put me on a fast track to success when I was very young, and I discovered I loved it there. I would accompany him to business meetings, where he often made me part of the discussions. I became comfortable in corporate settings.

As I grew up, my enterprising nature became more evident. Initially, I started a career in the photography business. Soon I was being given assignments to cover governors' balls and conventions, where I met many influential people. Even then, I knew how to be at ease in these situations. I could walk into a room of strangers and leave with new friends.

Photography was a fun, creative pursuit—but I had my eye on bigger things. That seed had been planted by my grandmother while I was still in high school. She lived in Jacksonville, Florida, and as we'd drive downtown, she would point to a skyscraper and say, "See that building right there?"

"Yes, ma'am."

"One day, Valerie, you're going to run a company like that. Be sure you keep your teeth and feet in good shape. Your feet to hold you up, and your teeth for a beautiful smile when you're on TV."

She was right. Ten years later I was well on my way. I was a top producer in a business investment firm after an influential businessman showed me the top arena of estate planning. When I discovered that many of my successful clients established important business relationships while playing golf, I learned to play. As a novice, I didn't realize that it was much more than just a game. I quickly learned that golf provided insight into a person's temperament and trustworthiness. Did they lie or cheat? How did they react to a bad shot? Were they calm and levelheaded or hotheaded? Were they impulsive, or did they think things through? As my game improved, I gained the respect and confidence of my fellow players. We had fun, told jokes, kidded around, and by the eighteenth hole we had a good idea of whether we would work well together.

I discovered that gaining a client's confidence and respect meant far more than titles or degrees. My father had taught me to look beyond elaborate presentations with slides and charts and to find out what a person really wants and needs.

In only a few short years, I was rewarded with a trip to Tahiti for being a top producer with one of the clients I represented. Among the award recipients, I was the youngest and the only woman.

At the ripe old age of twenty-four, I started my own company and, true to my nature, immediately set out to do what people said couldn't be done. In my business most agents work on commissions, but I had seen how this system didn't always benefit the client. I decided to forgo a commission, offering my clients, instead, a fee for my service, affording them more options and flexibility. This approach was well received by those who managed large portfolios and helped them to know the up-front costs, which are typically hidden.

I soon became known as a young pioneer. It presented me with so many opportunities that it wasn't long before I was running three companies. Trail-blazing has its challenges. Besides having unlimited opportunities, unexpected pitfalls may lie ahead. Resistance was fierce from my fellow estate planners, and I could see that I had forfeited the profit of hundreds of thousands of dollars in commissions when I chose to be fee-based rather than on commission. But forging ahead in uncharted waters energized me. Unfortunately, the energy I was expending was taking its toll.

As my business expanded, a personal challenge was exposed

in my work ethic. I found that I struggled with letting go and delegating. I felt the need to handle everything by myself. So there I was, juggling three companies, making every minute count to meet the needs of an ever-growing list of clients—all with little help. I worked long hours to be certain my clients' needs were met.

On September 16, 1995, I was at my office, finishing some reports so I could attend an evening networking event at the Orlando Chamber of Commerce. Suddenly I was overcome with a severe headache. It was like nothing I had ever experienced, and it was isolated on one side of my face. I turned the lights off in my office and lay my head on my desk, hoping that a power nap would help. But it didn't. The pain became so intense that my partner advised me just to go home.

I hoped to relax by taking a warm shower and then lying down for a little while before going to the Chamber of Commerce. I stepped into the shower and suddenly felt weightless, as though I were tumbling head over heels, like an astronaut in space. I could not discern which way was up, down, or sideways. My knees buckled, and I groped for the shower walls. I was surprised to discover that I was still upright as I felt like I was plummeting headfirst. Dizzy and nauseous from this sudden loss of equilibrium, I managed to open the shower door, grab a towel from the rack, and pull myself out of the shower. As I sank to the floor, I saw my portable phone on the top of the commode. I grabbed for it and dialed 911. The last thing I heard before losing consciousness was the operator's voice.

The sound of the fire rescue paramedics breaking in the front door roused me. There I was, lying on the bathroom floor buck naked, while two good-looking burly firemen stood over me. All I kept asking for was water.

"Ms. Greene, we're going to put you on a board and lift you onto a gurney," the firemen said.

Covering me with a warm blanket, they proceeded to lift me and place me on the gurney as promised. I was removed to the waiting ambulance.

The vomiting began shortly after I arrived in the emergency room. A nurse questioned me, but I had no idea what had happened to me or why. All I could tell her was that I had passed out in the shower.

"Dizzy, so dizzy," I kept repeating.

After six hours of tests, including an MRI, the results were given to me. The diagnosis was simple: "migrainous." I had never had a migraine before. I tried to relate to it as the kind of pain that my friends who suffered migraines must feel. An internist who was selected from my insurance plan wrote me a prescription for Inderal to treat the migraine and told me see her in two weeks. Tired and weak, I was sent home.

Two weeks later, I sat in the internist's office as she quickly glanced through my file, then let out a sigh. "Your MRI appears irregular, but these readings are so sensitive it's probably only a false positive. At your age you don't want something like that on your medical records. It would be too hard to get insurance."

I had heard of a false positive before. It's the medical way of saying that the test gave a wrong answer. I was relieved. Without ever explaining to me what she had seen on the MRI, the doctor told me to keep taking the Inderal.

I left her office with a funny feeling, however. As I walked down the hall, a name on a nearby door caught my attention. I knew Dr. Powers as a client. He was one of Orlando's leading neurosurgeons. I hesitated for a moment in front of his office and then, as if a hand on my back propelled me forward, I opened the door and walked in. Without planning to do so, I asked the receptionist, "Is Dr. Powers in?"

It was my lucky day. He was in.

"Val! Good to see you! What brings you in?" he asked. I told him what had happened, and about my false positive MRI. I read in his expression that he was concerned. After he examined me, he recommended that I have another MRI. Although I respected Dr. Powers's advice and had agreed to have another test, I was in no hurry to go through that claustrophobic and time-consuming procedure again. Besides, I had clients who needed me and a calendar full of appointments. So I put it out of my mind.

I continued to go to work daily, even though I felt extremely tired and lethargic, increasingly so each day. After a few more days of dragging myself to work, I came out of an appointment and told my business partner that I was too ill to work.

I drove home and went straight to bed. In the middle of the night I woke up with a piercing pain on the right side of my face, particularly in my jaw. The throbbing was so intense that it felt like my teeth were going to pop out. I later learned that although a stroke itself is not painful, the symptoms leading up to it are bizarre and often are excruciatingly painful. Had only I known then what I know now—my body was alerting me that something was terribly wrong. It knew what the doctors didn't know, and it was trying desperately to get my attention. It was telling me *Get to the hospital, now!* Instead I took another Inderal and went back to sleep.

By morning I was too weak to move. The right side of my body felt heavier than my left, and there was a constant, irritating buzzing in my ears. It was weeks before I was strong enough to walk, even around my house. During that time I slowly weaned myself off the Inderal, as I now suspected the drug may have been contributing to my weakness.

By November I was better. Although my right side was still weaker than my left, I was mobile and ready to put this episode behind me. I had enjoyed good health all my life, and being sick was foreign to me. I could hardly wait to jump back into my usual routine. To look at me, no one would ever imagine that I had suffered a stroke. After all, I was only thirty-one years old.

I scarcely gave the past two months a thought until the day I unexpectedly ran into Dr. Powers. He was concerned when I explained what had happened since I last saw him. As a neuro-surgeon, he couldn't treat me because I didn't need surgery, but he offered to call the neurologist who had reviewed my hospital tests and suggest that more tests be done.

"Would you send me your latest MRI film?" he asked. "I'm not comfortable with these episodes."

"Gregg, you know I hate that MRI machine," I complained. "It's frightening to be in that dark thing, and I'm claustrophobic."

"Okay, then go to Duran Medical Center, where they have an open MRI machine. The results won't be quite as detailed as the films from a closed MRI, but at least it will show me the basic picture."

This time I didn't hesitate. Within a week I went to the open MRI clinic and scheduled my test. After the tests were completed, I was lying in a hospital bed, patiently waiting for the results, when I heard Dr. Powers and a second physician discussing my case just outside my door.

"This new MRI shows a lesion that wasn't there on the previous one," Dr. Powers said. His voice was polite but urgent. "Due to the sudden onset, that lesion must have been caused by a stroke."

"I disagree; I believe it is MS," the other doctor insisted.

"But the sudden onset is true of a stroke, not MS."

"She has no risk factors for a stroke and she is too young," the second doctor replied.

I heard Dr. Powers excuse himself. Apparently the discussion was over. Soon the door to my room opened and a short, dark-haired man with a mustache walked over to my bed. At that time I had no way of knowing the important role he would soon play in my life.

"Hi, I'm Dr. Gonzalez." He shook my hand, then grabbed the side chair, swung it around, and straddled it. Resting his arm casually on the back of the chair, he flipped through the papers on his clipboard and began to explain what was wrong with me.

"Miss Greene, I have reviewed your latest test results. While there is a difference of opinion between myself and your friend Dr. Powers, as your neurologist I have concluded that you are suffering from the early stages of multiple sclerosis."

As he began to describe what that meant, I burst into tears. He waited a moment, and then told me that MS was aggravated by tension and stress. "I strongly advise you to take some time off from work. Why don't you go home and get some rest?"

Although this news was very upsetting, I began to think that Dr. Gonzalez might be right. I certainly had been under a lot of stress. *But why was Dr. Powers so insistent in his diagnosis of a stroke?* Fortunately, my career training included insurance underwriting, so I had all the resources I needed at home to satisfy my curiosity about this new diagnosis. On my return, I pulled out one of my medical books and studied up on stroke and multiple sclerosis. They did have similar symptoms, but the distinction between the two diseases was in the onset. I read that MS is a progressive disease that slowly deteriorates the myelin sheath around the nerves. Stroke, as the name implies, hits suddenly. *Dr. Powers had to be right.*

It was a great relief for me to think that multiple sclerosis was not in my future, but I still needed to follow Dr. Gonzalez's advice and take it easy for a while. My exhaustion had to be caused by something, and that something had to be stress. There was no other explanation. I asked my business partner to take over our shared work so I could spend a few months recuperating in Pensacola, where my older sister, Angie, and her husband lived with their seven-year-old son, Donnie. I would remain in Pensacola until I was ready to return to work.

Pensacola borders the Gulf of Mexico and is a charming, historical town with breathtaking views and snowy white beaches. It's called the Emerald Coast because of its crystal-clear, aqua-green water. Although it's a quiet place to raise a family, the pace of this small town was much too slow for Type

A me. Back home, I was busy nonstop. Here I had to work to find things to keep me occupied.

Angie's temperament was completely different from mine. She came to life very slowly in the morning as she fixed breakfast, packed Donnie's lunch, and drove him to school. In the evening we ate dinner around the dining room table and then watched TV in the family room by the fireplace. To me, Angie's life felt like a rerun of *Leave It to Beaver*.

In the meantime, I continued to wake up early, making a list of things to do that day. Before Angie had time to brush her teeth, I was knocking at her bedroom door, asking when we could go to the post office.

"Valerie, why on earth do you need to go to the post office? And why every day?"

"I need to mail some important letters," I answered.

I was bored; she was frustrated.

My exercise for the day was gathering twigs for the evening fire. When I couldn't find anything else to do, I would sit in a big easy chair with my Persian cat, Alex, nestled in my lap and read Angie's *Better Homes and Gardens*.

One cold day I was snuggled in front of the fire, skimming through yet another magazine, when an article, "Top Ten Neurologists in the United States," caught my attention. I read that one of them, a Dr. Rockwell, was practicing at the University of South Alabama, less than an hour from my sister's home in Pensacola. The article fired me up. I had to see this man. I had been evaluated by two neurologists and had two different opinions. I needed a third.

I was pretty sure it would be difficult to get an appointment with Dr. Rockwell, but after leaving a message with his staff, I received a call the next day. The doctor would see me, but first he wanted to review my MRI films. I arranged to have them sent to his office. I was thrilled! I had a purpose again! I was going to resolve the mystery of my illness.

After Dr. Rockwell completed a neurological evaluation, he

rejected the idea that I had MS and explained why he was convinced that I'd had a stroke. He recommended going to aquatic therapy to strengthen my weak side and to continue taking aspirin, as recommended by Dr. Powers. I was so relieved to hear confirmation that I did not have MS and was more determined than ever to get back to my busy life in Winter Park.

At the end of May, my friend Andy came to Pensacola, helped me pack my stuff into a U-Haul truck, and drove me home. I could hardly wait to get back to work. I was terribly disappointed, however, when I woke up the next day feeling tired and weak again. I thought I might have a touch of the flu. Having been gone so long, I didn't have any food in the house; and even though I didn't have an appetite, I knew I should eat something.

My next thought was of my grandmother, who lived nearby. She had always been there for me, and she was also well known for her southern cooking. One phone call and soon she and my grandfather were at my front door with a basket of food. My appetite miraculously returned when the comforting aromas filled the house—pot roast; potatoes; warm rolls; and, of course, something sweet for later.

She propped me up on the sofa with pillows in her familiar, caring way, and brought me a plate. Everything tasted delicious, but I was so tired that I could hardly hold the fork.

"Honey, I'm going to stay," she told me with a worried look on her face. I protested, but she insisted, then kissed my grandfather good night.

I was grateful that she stayed, as I grew worse during the night and woke up dizzy and nauseated. I wasn't going to take any more chances and told my grandmother that I needed to go to a hospital and be examined. A neighbor drove us, and my grandmother didn't leave my side. During the examination she grilled the doctor about his credentials, then asked him, "Do you have any children?"

"No, I'm single," he told her. While he turned to look at my chart, she arched her eyebrow and looked at me pointedly. She had always hoped that one day I'd marry a doctor. Meanwhile, I was trying to explain to him that I'd been to the hospital the previous fall with similar symptoms.

"Don't worry," he assured me with confidence. "We're going to run some tests and find out what's going on."

When he returned, he seemed intent on impressing us with his vast knowledge of the brain before his shared his diagnosis. "You have vertigo," he announced. "It's an inner ear infection that causes dizziness." He wrote me a prescription for Meclazine and sent me home.

The doctor was charming but very wrong! But he wasn't alone. Of the five doctors I had seen up to that point, three of them had misdiagnosed me. I didn't have vertigo. I didn't have MS. I didn't have a migraine. I had had a minor stroke. "Minor" can be deceptive because if you don't heed the warning, it can lead to a massive stroke. A blood clot would soon be heading for my brain, a silent killer on the loose, and my body was trying its level best to warn me. Ten days later, that clot reached my brain stem and nearly killed me.

It's a miracle that I survived.

Risk Factors

Up to 80 percent of strokes can be prevented.

—National Stroke Association

BEFORE MY FIRST STROKE, I didn't give this disease a thought. It was something that happened to other people, and no one close to me had gone through the experience. It's common not to think about a stroke until it happens—to yourself or to someone you love.

Still, in spite of the death and devastation caused by this disease, too many people ignore or aren't even aware of what those risks are. One out of three Americans can't even recognize the most common causes and symptoms of this disease, or knows about the three-hour window, or talks to their doctors about stroke at their annual checkup. That's why I call ignorance the number-one risk factor for stroke.

What you are about to read is pretty sobering. That's why I've begun this discussion of risk factors with the good news: stroke doesn't happen without cause. It can be prevented. We're not helpless onlookers. There are a lot of things we can do to avoid the tragedy of a massive brain attack. In fact, the early warning of a first stroke can turn out to be a big favor, as terrifying as it is, in providing people with the motivation they need to make necessary changes. Having experienced the devastation of a massive stroke, my motivation has been so strong that I've managed to prevent having another stroke for more than twelve years, day by day, by being very careful about how I treat myself and avoiding all the risks that can possibly be avoided.

How High Is Your Risk for a Stroke?

People at the highest risk for a stroke have one or more of the following, none of them by choice: high blood pressure (hypertension), atrial fibrillation (erratic heartbeat) or other forms of heart disease, a high cholesterol level, diabetes, and a family history of stroke. In addition, they *choose* to smoke, be sedentary and/or overeat, and drink alcohol excessively. If they have all of these risk factors, they are a stroke waiting to happen.

Following are statistical data on how much some of these major risk factors increase the likelihood of having a stroke.

- A blood pressure reading of 140/90 or higher: four to six times
- Heart disease: ten times
- A cholesterol level over 240: two times
- Cigarette smoking: two to three times
- Diabetes: two to four times
- Family history: two times
- Transient ischemic attack (TIA) or ministroke: ten times

Other Risk Factors

The conditions just mentioned are more widely recognized than a large number of other factors that contribute to stroke. Simply by being unknown increases the risk. In addition, a single risk factor may not increase a person's likelihood of having a stroke, but multiple risk factors will.

Age

Two out of three stroke victims are elderly. In spite of that statistic, older people are less aware of symptoms than are other groups. Brain imaging reveals that many elderly people have had an undiagnosed stroke.

Even though one out of three stroke victims are not elderly, youth is another risk factor. Still, there continues to be the widespread misperception that young people don't have strokes. They are also less likely to have health insurance and go for regular physical checkups, and are more likely to abuse drugs.

Illegal Drugs

Amphetamines, cocaine, and marijuana have been found to contribute to aneurysms and blood vessel malformations. In one study, 20 percent of the patients with an intracerebral hemorrhage had drugs in their system. Methamphetamine is toxic to large blood vessels and increases the risk of tears in major arteries in the neck.

Family History

Studies have shown that having a close relative, especially a father, who has suffered a stroke, is another risk factor, as are certain inherited disorders such as atrial fibrillation. Nevertheless, it's difficult to separate lifestyle choices from the genetic factor. If Dad was overweight, a heavy cigarette smoker, and ate a lot of bacon, those factors may be more of a warning than a genetic predisposition.

Geography

The Centers for Disease Control and Prevention studied the prevalence of stroke and found that the states with the highest rates of stroke were in the South, while the rate in northern states

Why Women Are at Special Risk

Stroke kills two and a half times more women than does breast cancer. Although more men have strokes than women, 62 percent of stroke deaths are women, and they also have worse long-term outcomes if they survive. Here are some facts behind these alarming statistics.

- Women are more likely than men to ignore symptoms.

- Women are less likely to call an ambulance.

- Women are more likely to report nontraditional symptoms, which may not be recognized as a stroke.

- Women are triaged more slowly in the emergency room.

- Women are less likely to get crucial tests and preventive treatments after an initial stroke.

- Women are two times more likely than men to have diabetes.

- Oral contraceptives and postmenopausal hormone replacement therapy are both risk factors for stroke.

- Pregnancy has been known to increase stroke risk.

- More women than men have migraine headaches, another risk factor for stroke.

- One out of five women does not know *any* of these risk factors for stroke.

A single factor may not be a major concern, but in combination they can be deadly. If a woman smokes, takes oral contraceptives, and has migraine headaches, her risk factor for stroke increases thirty-four times!

was lower. The author of the study attributed these differences to the prevalence of high stroke-risk factors in the South. Another factor is access to health care. There is a low number of hospitals with stroke centers in Mississippi, Arkansas, Oklahoma, Louisiana, and Alabama, the states with the highest prevalence of stroke.

Ethnicity

The ethnic group with the highest risk factor for stroke is Native Americans, followed by African Americans. These populations are also the least likely to live near a stroke center. One out of two African American women dies of stroke or heart-related disease.

Nevertheless, black people are more likely to survive a stroke than are white people, even though blacks have a higher rate of hypertension and diabetes. The survival rate for blacks five years after a stroke is 57 percent, as opposed to 36 percent for whites.

Stress

People who work in hospital rehab units are in a good position to note which occupations are common for stroke patients, and significant numbers are among those in high-stress occupations, such as executive officers, lawyers, and teachers. Yet stress does not appear on any of the lists of risk factors for stroke. When I told this to a speech pathologist, she said, "That just totally blows my mind." I am well aware of how severe stress contributed to the timing of my stroke, and I wonder why it isn't an "official" risk factor.

Many years ago stress was proven to cause the development of plaque in the bloodstream, a definite risk factor for stroke. A recent survey found that men who react intensely to situations that people normally regard as slightly stressful, such as being put on hold during a telephone call, had a higher incidence of stroke than men who didn't overreact to stress. Someone who constantly shouts "One more thing and I'm going to blow my top!" may not be far from the truth.

Depression

Depression is another emotional risk factor for stroke. People with severe depression were found to be 73 percent more likely to have a stroke than people who didn't report being depressed.

Because this list of risk factors may be bad news for a great many people, I want to repeat the good news from the National Stroke Association: *up to 80 percent of all strokes can be prevented.* Some can be eliminated on our own: the number-one risk factor in this category is cigarette smoking. If you smoke, are at high risk for a stroke, and value your life: quit. Hypertension, high cholesterol, atherosclerosis, carotid artery problems, atrial fibrillation, and diabetes can be treated or modified by a medical doctor, together with lifestyle change.

Ten Reasons for Seeing a Neurologist Right Away

One out of seven strokes is a recurring stroke. If this has happened to you, or if you are at high risk for a stroke, I strongly urge you to see a medical doctor, preferably a neurologist. Many advances have been made since I went from doctor to doctor after my stroke twelve years ago in an unsuccessful attempt to find out what was wrong with me. Getting a recommendation for a good neurologist is the best thing you can do for yourself at this point, because he or she will be familiar with the following breakthrough tests and treatments.

1. *ABCD score.* People who have had a TIA, or suspect they had one, need to see a neurologist within seven days after the symptoms occurred to take a simple test that has been found to be highly accurate in predicting another stroke. The acronym is based on an assessment of four factors: age, blood pressure, clinical features, and duration of symptoms.

The risk score will help physicians identify which patients should be given emergency treatment.

2. *Carotid endarterectomy.* New clinical practice guidelines have been issued by the American Academy of Neurology for treating the blockage or narrowing of a blood vessel in the carotid artery. It is the most commonly performed surgery for preventing stroke, and new studies show that it is often effective in treating patients who have recently had a TIA or experienced stroke symptoms.

3. *Inflammatory markers.* Researchers have found that high levels of two proteins in the blood of stroke survivors are strong indicators of a recurring stroke. These tests determine the levels of C-reactive protein (CRP) and lipoprotein-associated phospholipase A2 (LpPLAZ) that help doctors identify patients who need treatment. A high level of CRP is a predictor of a severe stroke. It indicates an urgent need for aggressive treatment and the elimination of risk factors through lifestyle changes.

4. *Atrial fibrillation (AF).* Recent studies show that this high-risk condition for stroke has been successfully treated with warfarin (Coumadin), an anticoagulant, in more than two out of three patients. A large comparison study of different treatments for atrial fibrillation suggests that warfarin is the most beneficial, both for patients who are currently experiencing AF and for those who have a history of irregular heartbeat.

5. *Homocysteine.* A high concentration of this amino acid in the blood has been identified as a possible risk factor for stroke, and early studies have resulted in further trials to rule out the contribution of other factors, such as smoking. Homocysteine levels can be lowered by taking folic acid and B vitamins as precautionary measures.

6. *Retinopathy (eye blood vessel damage).* A change in the small blood vessels in the eye has been found to be a risk

factor for stroke. By studying photographs of changes in the blood vessels in the retina, researchers found that patients with blood vessel damage were 70 percent more likely to have a stroke than patients without damage.

7. *Silent brain lesions.* A recent study has shown the importance of having an MRI scan after a first stroke. Changes in tissue in scans taken within three months following a stroke help doctors identify new lesions, indicating the death of brain cells that have occurred *without symptoms* since the stroke. These are an indication of a blockage or reduction of blood flow to the brain, a condition that must be treated to prevent the recurrence of stroke.

8. *fMRI.* This new diagnostic tool is also showing neuroscientists how the brain works to repair motor function that has been damaged by stroke, shedding light for the first time on the brain's ability to reorganize neural pathways between the hemispheres. By imaging the brains of patients shortly after the stroke occurred and again several months later, they were able to track the progress of brain reorganization while patients performed tasks with their weakened hand. The fMRI has been found to be a valuable tool in improved diagnosis, treatment, and recovery from a stroke. Discuss it with your neurologist for updates, and ask whether any new developments might be useful in treating you.

9. *Two biomarkers that predict recurring stroke.* A study in patients who had an ischemic stroke has identified a molecule (sVCAM-1) and a peptide (NT-proBNP) that assist doctors in determining the risk level of another attack and methods for preventing it.

10. *"Triple therapy" drugs.* The amount of brain damage caused by a stroke has been found to be reduced when a combination of aspirin, cholesterol drugs, and blood pressure drugs was given to patients who came to the hospital within twenty-four hours after the onset of a stroke. Discuss with

your neurologist how this treatment might benefit you in the event of a recurrence.

In addition to encouraging you to see a neurologist, I also urge anyone at high risk for a stroke or a recurring stroke to see a holistic physician. I highly recommend the treatments I received, which are explained in detail in the section "Integrative Medicine" in chapter 8, "In the Crucible of Change."

3

Acute Care

―――――――――

IHAVE BEEN TOLD that denial is the first stage of grief, and that was my experience as well. Perhaps it serves as a buffer, holding at arm's length a reality too overwhelming for the mind to take in all at once. I comforted myself in those first days following the stroke by refusing to believe that I was paralyzed. Try as I might to deceive myself about the gravity of my condition, my body was weak. I was exhausted. Who wouldn't be—lying there as I was—hooked up to endless wires and tubes, loud, beeping monitors, my sleep constantly interrupted by nurses who poked and prodded me in the middle of the night?

I was so hypersensitive to noise that the rattling of food carts or the distant sound of people talking would awaken me. Alarmed and anxious, I was unable to fall back to sleep without a struggle. Then, just as I started dozing off, I'd be blinded by bright lights turned on by the lab technician for another blood drawing. Those were not easy, as my veins were small and difficult to find. I decided that the last place on earth for a person to get rest was while in a hospital. I just needed to go home, I reassured myself. Then everything would be all right.

The day after my massive stroke, I woke to the sound of voices softly harmonizing. My mother and grandparents had gathered around my bed and filled my room with the melodious sound of sacred hymns being sung. A friend, Dr. Bill Spain, also was there. He had flown down from Pensacola to see me. Bill is one of the most charismatic human beings I know, and his presence could lighten the atmosphere of any space. I wrote a note and handed it to him, and he understood right away what I needed.

"Come on," he said, "let's sing something more spirited." Respectfully, my family followed his lead and joined in an upbeat rendition of a livelier psalmody.

Add to this mix my good friend Andy, who then appeared at my door, carrying a duffel bag and wearing a mischievous smile.

"I've brought someone who misses you," he said with a grin. He gently placed the duffel bag on the bed, opened the bag, and a little furry black head popped out. It was Alex! I burst

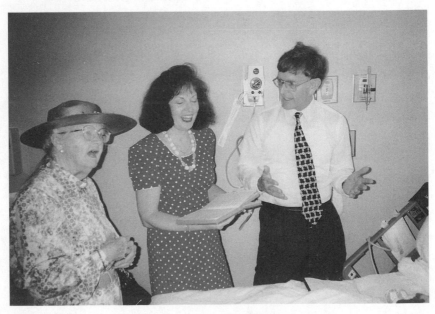

My grandmother and mother with Dr. Bill Spain

into tears of joy. Andy knew how much I loved my cat, and he had secreted him past security. My beloved Alex lay on my chest and purred loudly. Cats just have a way of knowing what you need, especially my Alex.

I was grateful for all the company, but the visit had exhausted me. My eyes closed. It was too much of an effort to keep them open. The voices faded to a dim hum as I began to nod off. I heard a nurse's voice, then silence. The visit was over. Even more than the comfort provided by family and friends, my body and especially my damaged brain needed the healing powers of sleep.

On the fifth morning in the hospital I woke up, startled. My bed was moving! I looked around and realized I was being wheeled down the hall. *Where was I going now?* Not being able to speak was terrifying and heightened these moments of help-lessness when I had no control over my circumstances.

"Everything's okay, honey," said a nurse. "There's nothing to worry about. We're taking you to your own room."

Hallelujah! I was finally making progress.

Once I was settled into my new room, I felt much better, so grateful to be unhooked from those loud monitors of the ICU. Once again I thought about how Dr. Gonzalez had told me I was paralyzed. Nonsense, I reasoned. The doctor was simply wrong again. I decided that the only way to know for sure was to find out for myself. The solution was simple: I'd get out of bed and stand up! That would put an end to all this pessimism and negativity.

Slowly I scooted over to the edge of the bed, my right side dragging my numb and lifeless left side behind it. This was not an easy maneuver, but I was determined to make it, inch by inch. Finally I reached the edge, lowered my right leg, braced myself with my right arm, and gave myself a little push. Immediately I lost my balance and fell to the floor. My left side felt like heavy Jell-O. As I lay there, frightened and scarcely able to move, I took in, for the first time, the doctor's words that I had previously refused to believe: *You are paralyzed.*

I lay on the floor for several minutes, terrified by my helplessness, until a nurse passed by and saw me.

"Oh, my God, child, what have you done?"

I opened my mouth to explain but, of course, nothing came out. She lifted me up and helped me back into bed. It was obvious by the look on her face that she was concerned about my state of mind. "I'm going to call your doctor."

Minutes later, a doctor came in and immediately began asking me questions.

"Do you know where you are?" I nodded, then motioned for my pen and paper as the questions kept coming:

"Who is the president of the United States?"

"What year is it?"

I had no difficulty writing down my answers, but I did wonder why he was asking me all these silly questions. It was only later that I realized he was trying to determine whether I had lost any of my mental faculties, such as my memory or the ability to understand what people were saying. Although patients often suffer these losses poststroke, I was fortunate. I did, however, struggle with comprehension—which was evident in how mystified I was by his asking so many questions of me. I honestly could not reason what possible purpose he had in asking questions of me that a child could answer.

My friend Andy walked into the room during the questioning, and the doctor asked me, "Do you know who he is?"

I smiled and wrote the name "Elvis." The doctor looked shocked. I must be worse off than he'd thought! Andy laughed as he explained that Elvis was a nickname I'd given him because he once lived near Graceland, Elvis Presley's mansion in Tennessee. Though I had lost much, thank God I hadn't lost my sense of humor!

To be sure, my brain was firing all its pistons; however, the doctor continued to ask me more questions. Apparently he was satisfied with my mental acumen, because he then proceeded to run a needle lightly along my face and down the left side of my body to the bottom of my foot.

"Do you feel any sensation?" he asked.

I shook my head, shocked and bewildered, because I felt nothing.

"Can you move the fingers and toes on your left side?"

No problem. I can do that! But when I went to move, I could not believe my own eyes. They would not move! *This can't be happening to me!* I felt as though I were watching a scene out of a movie; it was surreal. *This must be happening to someone else!*

"The next step for you is rehabilitation," the doctor told me. "You need physical therapy."

"How soon?" I scrawled, encouraged by the thought that something could be done about my immobility.

"As soon as your insurance approves it," he replied. "We've already contacted your insurance carrier to let them know you need rehab. Unfortunately, approval can take several days."

While the doctor wrote in my chart, my mind was going a mile a minute, putting together a plan to expedite my transfer to rehab. My friend Herb handled my health insurance. We had worked together at the first investment and insurance firm I represented. Herb was tall, handsome, sharply dressed, and a real go-getter, and he and I quickly connected and became friends. Being the youngest reps in an all-white, all-male firm, we laughingly referred to ourselves as the "token" duo—a black man and a woman. After I left the firm to start my own business, I encouraged Herb to do the same. Taking a giant leap of faith, he started an insurance agency that had grown into one of the most successful in the state of Florida.

As soon as the doctor left, I wrote a note to Andy, asking him to call Herb. I was relieved and comforted to know that I had a friend and a powerful insurance agent who could help me get into rehab as soon as possible.

Later that afternoon, a group of friends came to cheer me

up. They brought a large get-well poster, which they had all signed, and hung it over my bed and took turns saying a few words of encouragement. I was grateful for their company, but I was also very embarrassed. Unable to hold my neck up, the left side of my face drawn down and drooping, I was not a pretty sight. My hair was a fright, and I wore no makeup. The well-groomed and put-together woman they had known was now drooling and unable to speak. They tried to mask their fear and pity, but I could read it in their faces. I looked pathetic.

After they left, I began making plans again, as was my nature. *This isn't who I am!* I had to get out of that hospital as soon as possible. I had to get into rehab, go through recovery, and get back to work. As soon as Andy returned, I wrote him another note: "Call Herb!"

"We already called him," Andy said.

"Call again!" I wrote.

The stroke had traumatized my nervous system so severely that the least little thing could set off intense frustration, exacerbating my already impatient nature. It had been only an hour since Andy had first called Herb. Even so, several times that day and the next, he willingly called Herb every time I asked him to find out what progress had been made with my insurance company.

The trauma to my brain caused by the stroke could wreak havoc on my behavior. At times I was lucid and logical, but at other times I would become completely agitated and upset at the smallest things. I'll never forget how upset I became over a piece of pie that was wrong. I love banana cream pie and had requested a slice from a specific bakery. However, the pie I was brought was lemon. This upset me terribly, and I began to cry. I was so hurt by the error, I could not control my emotions.

Angie can attest to my bizarre behavior as one day she came to the hospital and found me highly agitated, trembling in my bed. I handed her a note that read: "They're trying to kill me!"

"What?"

"In the showers," I wrote. A shock of fright went through me at the thought of that large, cold, tiled room; of having to sit again in that plastic shower chair with the hollow seat, naked and shivering, waiting for the water to be turned on.

"What on earth do you mean?" My sister's eyes went wide.

I couldn't understand why she was just standing there when I was in such danger. Frantic, I grabbed the pen and wrote in big letters: "NAZIS!"

She left with a disturbed look on her face and walked to the nurses' station, where she asked politely, "Could I see where my sister is getting her showers?"

As I was waiting for her to return, so terrified I could scarcely breathe, I heard Angie and a nurse having a conversation outside my door. The nurse explained to her that after a stroke, many patients' memories get stirred up. She described it as a file cabinet that has fallen over. "All the file folders and papers are scattered on the floor. The information is there, but it's not in order and cannot be easily retrieved. Hopefully, in time your sister will be able to reorganize all those files."

I tried very hard to comprehend this information, but it just made me more confused. When Angie came in the room she told me in a reassuring voice, "The showers are fine. I checked them out carefully. You don't have to be afraid."

"Please, please, take me home!" I wrote.

"Val, you know I can't do that. But you can trust these nurses. They understand."

It was only later that I could make sense of the powerful feelings of terror and humiliation I had experienced in the showers. They had become scrambled with a scene from a Holocaust documentary I had seen years before in which terrified, naked people in a similar large, tiled room were about to be gassed to death. But I didn't know at the time that my brain was busy trying to reorganize the files that had been scattered by my stroke. To me, the threat in the hospital shower room was real.

．　．　．

During the day, Angie, Andy, and my mom took turns staying with me. They would press the "call" button near my bed when I needed assistance, a nurse would respond, and they would tell her what I needed. But at night, and sometimes during the day, I was by myself. One afternoon when I was alone, I urgently needed to use the bathroom. Without thinking much about it, I pressed the call button myself with my good hand and waited.

"Yes?" said a voice.

I tried to force air through my vocal cords, but nothing came out. The only thing I could think of was to press the call button again.

"Yes?" came the voice again, but it was too late. I had wet the bed.

"Do you need something?"

Again I tried to respond. I had never felt so helpless and humiliated. I lay in that urine-soaked sheet for quite a while until Andy arrived. Embarrassed, I wrote him a note explaining what had happened. He immediately called for a nurse.

After she changed the sheets, the nurse put a plastic pad under me and in a matter-of-fact voice told me, "If it happens again, just wet the bed."

No way! I thought. I wanted to scream, "Do you have any idea what it feels like to be so helpless, so humiliated?"

She must have read my thoughts by the anguished look on my face, because she assured me that she'd tell all the nurses on the shift to respond in person whenever I pressed the call button. "But if we're all busy and can't get here in time, it will be easier for us to change this pad than to change the whole bed."

I had no choice but to let the plastic pad stay, but it horrified me. It was so degrading. Little did I know that this indignity would be the first of many. I lay there in my misery and the fear that my life would never be the same.

The next morning, a woman came to my room with a wheel-chair. "Ms. Greene, your insurance company has approved inpatient rehabilitation, and I'm here to take you to your new room in the rehab wing."

Yes! You did it, Herb! I felt such relief as the therapist wheeled me down the corridors, my zest for living having returned. *I can do this!* I was athletic, my strength would come back, and I'd be out of rehab in no time—and then I could go home. At that moment, I had no idea I would be in the hospital for more than a month.

"Here we are," the therapist said as the wheelchair came to a stop. I stared in amazement at the room number—1481—the same as in my home street address. How extraordinary! However, in my confused state of mind, I was sure the nurses had chosen this room on purpose to make me feel at home. Years later I realized it was one of those serendipitous moments in life that encourage us and keep us on our path.

I settled in and surveyed my room. It had a big window with a view of the grounds leading to the parking lot, which was nice, but from my bed, all I could see was the side of a brick wall. The room was furnished with standard hospital decor: bed, nightstand, dresser, white walls on which hung a TV, a clock, a calendar, and a bulletin board listing my therapy schedule—certainly not the best environment to cheer a person up. At times it felt more like a prison cell with its cold, barren walls.

I lay in that bed, decorating those bare walls in my mind with some of my photography, and tried to cheer up. I comforted myself realizing that things were moving ahead. Pretty soon I'd have my life back. All I had to do was follow that schedule on the bulletin board and work, work, work, just as I had done during my early morning workouts in the gym for years. My eyes fell onto the wall calendar, and I was surprised to find out it was the eighteenth of June. I thought of the daily planner on my desk and the long lists of tasks to do and clients to call each day. *Would I ever return to work? And what about driving? Oh, my God, would I ever drive again?* Pretty soon my mind was racing with thoughts about my future until I was overwhelmed with anxiety.

That night, in the dark silence of my room, my loneliness became unbearable. As I lay in a fetal position, taking in the enormity of all that had happened to me, I began sobbing. No sound came forth, only tears. One of the night nurses came into my room, somehow knowing I needed comforting. She sat on the edge of my bed and rubbed my back with baby powder until I fell fast asleep. I will never forget her. She was one of those angels who come into our lives, without bidding, at moments when they are needed most.

I woke up the next morning having to use the bathroom, pressed the call button, and waited.

"Yes?" came a voice. But no one came. I pressed the call button again, waiting for her response even longer this time.

"Yes?" came the voice again. *Didn't she know I couldn't respond?*

Still no one came. There was no way I was going to lie there and wet the bed. I waited a little longer before deciding I was now strong enough to crawl to the bathroom. But I wasn't. While sliding off the bed, I fell and cut my face on the bedside table. Hearing the crash, the nurses came on the run. When Angie arrived at lunch, I was sitting on the edge of the bed with my face bandaged. She was livid when she read my note, explaining what had happened, and she filed a complaint. After that, the nurses responded in person.

Angie had brought a videotape about me that had been aired in Pensacola by my friend Dr. Spain, who hosted a live TV show on health. Angie reserved the rehab VCR and invited several of my nurses to watch it with us. During the broadcast Dr. Spain showed a photo of me with Angie, described my stroke, and asked his viewers to pray for me and send cards to my room. I cried when I saw the photo, remembering how vibrant and vivacious I looked. That beautiful businesswoman in the photograph looked so confident and proud. Now who was I?

"Wow! Look how pretty you are!" said the nurses. I knew their intentions were good, but it was the kind of praise you would lavish on a young child. I was insulted. Although in many ways I had to become like a little child again, my trauma-tized brain was unable to perceive that.

Fear and frustration were my constant companions. As I started doing things for myself, challenges consumed my every effort. Although it was a relief to be taken to the bathroom instead of using a bedpan, each trip was exhausting. My leg and trunk muscles were so weak that I had to hold on to a nurse as she lowered me slowly to the toilet. Before she left, she made sure I knew how to pull the red "help" cord hanging from the wall when I needed her to come back and lift me up.

Everything was hard work. Even simple tasks such as brush-ing my teeth and tying my tennis shoes for rehab were tedious and time-consuming. Using only one hand may not seem to be much of a problem until you have no other alternative. As for trying to keep up my appearance, I started wearing a baseball cap on my bad-hair days, which were pretty much every day. Thank God there wasn't a mirror in my room. I'd glimpsed my drooping face in a bathroom mirror once and didn't look again. It was scary.

But my clothing was another matter. Upon entering the business world I had been very discerning about my appear-ance, always dressing for success, and I wasn't going to lower my standards just because I was in the hospital. When I was able to wear my own clothes, Angie brought several of my comfortable and cute fitness outfits from my home that were perfect for rehab. She neatly arranged the pants with their coordinating tops in the dresser. The nurse who dressed me for my first day in rehab must have been too busy to notice that the top she put on me had a black striped pattern that didn't match the polka dot pattern of the pants. I didn't say anything at the time, but I became increasingly agitated over my mis-matched outfit.

When Angie arrived, I wrote her a note asking her to help me change my clothes. She read my note and asked, "What's wrong with what you're wearing? You look fine."

I bristled as I pointed to the two patterns. She had to look twice before she noticed that they weren't the same.

"Oh, good grief, Val!" Angie exclaimed. "They look fine together. The difference is hardly noticeable! But I'll change you if that will make you happy!"

One of my rehab nurses stopped in as she was putting on the correct pants, and Angie asked her if they could chat in the hallway. I listened closely to their conversation.

"She has the strangest fears," my sister was saying. "She gets so frustrated over the smallest things."

"That's totally normal," the nurse assured her. "Valerie's been traumatized by the stroke, but she's one of the lucky ones. Her memory and cognitive functions are returning, but she's incredibly frustrated because she can't tell us what she needs. Her extreme sensitivity is perfectly normal at this stage. She'll be fine. Just give her some time."

From then on, the nurses made sure that my clothes were coordinated.

After my early-morning showers and the challenges of getting dressed, I would be so fatigued that I just wanted to go back to bed. Instead, another therapist arrived to feed me my pureed breakfast and monitor my swallowing function. All my food had to be mashed or blended because my throat muscles were so weak I could barely swallow. I couldn't even have a glass of water for fear of it being aspirated into my lungs. Instead, a substance called Thicken was added that turned liquids into a gelatinous substance within seconds. When I used to work out, I had downed many energy shakes that weren't too tasty, but this stuff was just gross. When we were children, my father teased my sisters and me by asking if we wanted a cup of mud. This was pretty darn close!

Once a week, "swallow studies" and X-rays were made of my throat to monitor changes. I graduated from pureed foods to soft foods such as oatmeal, applesauce, and mashed potatoes, and then to solids such as bananas. I advanced quickly and was ready to have my meals with my fellow patients.

I was horrified, however, on what I encountered on my first morning in the gathering room. The room was filled with brain-injury patients, mostly stroke survivors, although some had suffered either severe car accidents or sports injuries. One young man had been kicked in the head while playing soccer and wore a halo with screws in his head. Ouch! It gave me the willies just to look at him. We all sat, expressionless, strapped securely in our wheelchairs, slumped to one side. I lost my appetite watching everyone drooling saliva and food uncontrollably. To my dismay, I realized I was in the same condition.

After breakfast and a short break, I was wheeled to the gym for physical therapy. It was unlike any gym I had ever seen, filled with large colored balls, matted tables, and walkers. I was wheeled over to one of the matted tables and introduced to Christine, a young woman with long blond hair who would be my physical therapist for the next few weeks. She helped me out of my wheelchair and onto the table. I lay on my back while she assessed the condition of my leg and arm. While she took notes, I looked around and saw a patient with one leg learning to walk and others struggling to do the simplest tasks. Hanging my head in despair, I wondered how I was ever going to overcome my condition.

The thirty-minute session with Christine was emotionally draining. I wanted to leave; no, I wanted to crawl into a hole and die. Instead, I was wheeled around the corner to speech therapy. This room wasn't much bigger than a broom closet.

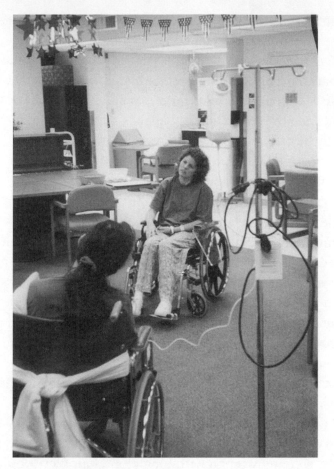

Me in wheelchair

"Hi, I'm Beth, your speech therapist," said a woman younger than me with light auburn hair. Friendly and eager, she was ready to get going. Not me. I was overwhelmed and could hardly concentrate. All I could focus on was what I had lost. This once dynamic woman was now reduced to living in half her body. Couldn't speak. Couldn't even make sounds. I was still in there, but no one could hear me. It was like being buried alive.

.   .   .

I fell into a deep depression, refusing to leave my room, barely able to eat. At night I had a recurring nightmare of being inside a casket, trying to scream as I was lowered into the ground. Terror at the sound of clods of dirt hitting the casket jolted me awake, chest pounding, covered in sweat, and afraid of going back to sleep.

Angie became very concerned. By nature she is nurturing and full of compassion, but she gets frustrated when she can't make things better. When she first started realizing the extent of my paralysis, she would urge me to "just be a patient." She wanted me to lie there and be taken care of. My sister was so happy and relieved that I was alive that she was okay with me lying in a bed with food rolling down my face. As she came to grasp the depth of my depression and grief over what I had lost, she did everything she could think of to cheer me.

"Just be glad you're here," she insisted. "You don't need to be the perfect Val."

"I'd rather be dead," I wrote.

I saw the hurt look on her face, but that was how I felt. I had a completely different perspective from hers. She was willing to settle for less. I was not.

The nurses also were concerned over my state of mind. They called the rehab doctor, who prescribed a session with a psychologist. For some reason three showed up. I must have been in really bad shape, a case study or something, to qualify for a private session with three shrinks. They came into my room somber and professional, one wearing a cute paisley bow tie. The "leader" began to speak in a sympathetic yet condescending manner.

"Ms. Greene—Valerie—we understand how difficult and frustrating this must be for you. We are here to offer our assistance as you work through accepting your limitations."

Limitations! I'm not accepting any limitations. And how on earth can you even begin to understand? As my indignation grew, it sparked a fire that began to blaze deep within me.

Didn't they realize that the woman lying like a lump in her bed was not the woman I really was? I motioned for my writing board, which they quickly handed to me, eager to understand how I felt.

Searching for a way to express myself, a name flashed through my mind: Lorena Bobbitt. Earlier that year she had been on the national news. After discovering that her husband was cheating on her, she had cut off his penis, took it for a drive, and threw it out the window into a vacant lot. Amazingly, his penis was found and surgically sewn back on. The reattachment was so successful that he became a pornographic film star. He even went on talk shows, where he was celebrated as an example of the miracles of modern medicine.

I wrote furiously, in capital letters, and then turned my board to face the three doctors. It read: IF THEY CAN FIX BOBBITT'S DICK, THEY CAN FIX ME!!

I've never seen a group of doctors so stunned. They just stood there. After a long silence they left, one of them snickering. I think they got the point. I was much more alert than they had assumed, and they realized that I wasn't going to accept *any* limitations.

Most important was that I now realized it, too. My anger had awakened my fighting spirit, igniting that fire within. As my heart pounded, I promised myself that I would do everything in my power to recover. Clearly, I couldn't depend on the doctors alone to change my situation. It would need my involvement, too. I would bring my personal best to the work of rehab, and I would search for health care professionals who didn't buy into the idea of accepting limitations but believed I could recover fully. My depression vanished, burned away by my determination. It was true I'd had a stroke, but it didn't have me!

Listen here, I told my stroke, *you picked the wrong girl!*

Word of the incident with the three doctors traveled fast through the hospital corridors. One of the older nurses came to my room and told me, "Honey, you are going to be fine. You're a fighter. The quiet, complacent patients are the ones we worry about."

I returned to rehab with a vengeance, where the therapists and nurses were excited by my transformation. All my life I had been told that a mustard seed of faith could move mountains. With my faith restored, it was time to start moving mountains!

When the Crisis Is Over:
For the Family

*I go in and out of consciousness, and, yet, I feel fully alert.
There are so many streams of thoughts which run through
my mind. Will I live to discover new mysteries and find these
truths which God has created? Have I been able to provide
a stone to this edifice of knowledge? I can only hope.*

—Louis Pasteur, 1868, shortly after his stroke

NO MATTER WHAT has happened, there's hope. In the aftermath of a massive stroke, when loved ones are still in shock and confused and when reality is beginning to set in, two things are important to remember: the brain is an amazingly resilient survivor, and no two strokes are alike. No one can accurately predict how much recovery will take place.

At age forty-five, Louis Pasteur suffered a massive stroke that paralyzed his entire left side—*before* he made his most important discoveries. As the quotation at the beginning of this section shows, the stroke did not affect his mental capacities at all. Years later, his discovery of immunization did much more than "provide a stone to this edifice of knowledge"; it also revolutionized the field of medicine. But Pasteur couldn't have known what the future held for him in the terrifying aftermath of his stroke. At that time, all he could rely on was a single word: hope.

This is not to deny that a massive stroke is a catastrophic, life-altering event for all involved, but I also have experienced the power of hope. That's why the single most important thing that you can do right now for the patient—and for yourselves—is not to buy into anyone's negativity. Although no one knows what the future will bring, studies show that the extent of recovery is influenced by the strength of the patient's network of support provided by family and friends.

I am aware of the enormity of such a responsibility, and at the moment you may not feel up to taking it on, but there's no more paralyzing burden than hopelessness. My advice is to let go of the future. What's important is today. You most likely felt completely helpless during the crisis, but once it has passed and the survivor has been stabilized, you can play an active role in achieving the best possible outcome.

A Crash Course in Medical Terms

I have received hundreds of phone calls from people whose loved ones have survived a stroke, and from them I have learned that the two things they need most from the hospital staff are compassion and information. The state of medical care today is pretty crazy: doctors and nurses are understaffed and underpaid, while hospital administrators are paid too much, and health insurance companies, not physicians, determine what kind of tests and treatments can be given. In such a work situation, empathy may be in short supply. You have no control over that pressing need, but you do have control over the kind of information you receive.

As you flag down doctors rushing off to treat the next patient, asking them to explain "What's an infarction?" is wasting valuable time. Because they don't have the luxury of giving you a lesson in Neurology 101, the information you receive may leave you more bewildered than you were before. If there ever was a time when you need to educate yourself about the terminology of stroke care, it's now. The more knowledgeable you are, the better the quality of information the hospital staff can give you. The following sections briefly explain terms and procedures related to acute stroke care.

Locating the Damage

After the patient has been stabilized, the next step is to detect where and what type of stroke has taken place. The area where brain cells have died is called an *infarction*. It appears on a scan as a well-defined *lesion*. Around it are tissues that have been weakened by the stroke but are not dead. This area is called an *ischemic penumbra*, and while the dead tissues are a lost cause, the cells in the penumbra are not functioning but can be reactivated in a number of ways that you will learn about later in this book.

The value of the CT scan explained in chapter 1 is that it quickly rules out a bleed, but other imaging tools accurately pinpoint the type of stroke that has occurred, the part of the brain it has affected, and the extent to which brain cells have died.

- *Magnetic resonance imaging (MRI)* is usually not given during the three-hour window after the onset of a stroke, when every minute counts. An hour is required to obtain MRI results, and they don't give a clear picture of the anatomy of the brain if patients don't remain perfectly still during the scan—an impossibility if they are vomiting or having seizures. In special cases, it may be necessary to give an MRI during that time, because it is superior to a CT scan in detecting the presence or the absence of an ischemic stroke. After the crisis has passed, an MRI becomes an important tool in evaluating the extent of the damage.

- *Diffusion-weighted imaging (DWI)* is an advanced diagnostic tool, the most powerful to date, which is likely to be available only at fully equipped stroke centers. It can detect where damage is taking place in the early stages of stroke development, before the forming of lesions. With very aggressive treatment given early, it can prevent the death of brain cells. It can even detect a TIA.

- *Angiography* is a video X-ray of the arteries that supply the brain, and for a long time it was the gold standard for detecting the whereabouts of a clot, but (as in my case) it has become the method of last resort because of the dangers involved. The catheter that is inserted in a vessel in the groin can cause bleeding or dislodge the blockage, and patients also can have an allergic reaction to the dye used during the procedure.

- *Computed tomography angiography (CTA)* uses a CT scanner with special software. Although it is less invasive, safer, and produces images in minutes, it is not as precise as an angiogram.

- *Magnetic resonance angiography (MRA)* is another advanced diagnostic tool. Safe, noninvasive, and similar to an MRI, it provides clear images of the arteries in the brain as well as other arteries that deliver blood to the brain.

- *Carotid ultrasound* detects any narrowing of the carotid arteries by placing an instrument over the patient's neck, or in the ophthalmic artery by placing it over the patient's closed eye.

- *Electroencephalogram (EEG)* records electrical abnormalities in the brain that cause seizures, the violent, involuntary contractions of muscles that are common after a stroke.

- *Transcranial doppler (TCD)* is a bedside test in which a probe is placed against the skull. It can identify blockage and monitor the flow of blood in the brain after treatment has begun, measuring its progress.

- *Positron-emission tomography (PET) scan* indicates the condition of brain tissue, which may be functioning even though there is a reduction of blood flow, and helps identify injuries the stroke may have caused.

- *Electrocardiogram (ECG)* is used to evaluate the electrical current in the heart.
- *Echocardiogram* is used to find blood clots in the heart that can travel to the brain, causing another stroke.

Types of Ischemic Stroke

When the test results come back, you will be confronted with another avalanche of terms, depending on the kind of stroke that has occurred. If the patient has suffered an ischemic attack, blood flow to the brain has been blocked in one of the two major arterial systems.

- The *carotid arteries* are located on the front of the neck to either side of the brain stem. You can feel their pulse by gently placing a finger and thumb under your jaw.
- The *basiliar* is a single artery in the brain stem, directly under the skull. The arteries of the vertebrae join there and become one. The kind of stroke I had was a blockage of the basiliar (also called basal) artery.

The kind of clot—and its origin—that is responsible for an ischemic stroke is of three types:

- *Thrombotic.* This stroke occurs when a clot *(thrombus)* forms in an artery that has become hardened *(artherosclerosis)* by a buildup of cholesterol or plaque. The stroke occurs when the clot closes up the narrow passageway, shutting off the blood supply.
- *Embolic.* This type of stroke is caused by plaque or a blood clot that has become dislodged in an artery in the heart or another artery that supplies blood to the brain and then travels to the brain. Some embolic strokes are caused by

atrial fibrillation, an abnormal rhythm of a heartbeat that causes blood to remain in a chamber of the heart where it forms a clot that dislodges and travels to the brain.

- *Lacunar.* These are a series of very mild ischemic strokes that warn of the possibility of a major stroke. Symptoms are sudden weakness, stumbling, or other clumsiness. As the symptoms are mild and can be attributed to other causes, they are often not identified as a stroke.

Treatment of Ischemic Stroke

Surgical treatments include an *embolectomy*, the removal of the lesion caused by an embolism. Another surgical procedure is a *carotid endarterectomy.* If the walls in the carotid artery are rigid and thick, a condition called *stenosis,* they can become so narrow that blood flow to the brain is reduced. In severe cases, this may require a surgical procedure that cleans out the plaque on the inside of the artery wall. Although there is a risk of heart attack or another stroke from having this surgery, it results in improved motor function, speech, and vision impaired by the stroke.

A number of drugs are used as anticlotting measures in treating an ischemic attack. One group treats blood platelets, which stick together and cause blood clotting. Aspirin is the most common. Other antiplatelet drugs, such as clopidogrel (Plavix), are known as *thienopyridines glycoprotein inhibitors*.

Another group of drugs is called anticoagulants, which thin the blood. *Warfarin* (Coumadin) is important in treating patients with atrial fibrillation and others who can't take antiplatelets. It does increase the risk of bleeding, however, and the FDA has strengthened its warning of that potential side effect.

Heparin has been another anticoagulant drug of choice for decades, but it is also going out of favor because a number of recent studies show that it is no more effective than aspirin while it increases the risk of a hemorrhagic stroke. *Direct thrombin inhibitors* (DTIs), derived from natural sources, is a new class of anticoagulants that is effective and poses less of a risk of bleeding. *Atorvastin* (Lipitor) is an anticholesterol drug that reduces the risk of another stroke.

Types of Hemorrhagic Stroke

Although hemorrhagic strokes account for less than 20 percent of all strokes, they are responsible for 30 percent of all stroke deaths. The cause is most commonly a history of hypertension, which weakens blood vessels. When a rupture finally occurs, blood spills into the brain, putting dangerous amounts of pressure on the delicate tissues of the brain, destroying neurons and blood vessels. Following are the major types of hemorrhagic stroke:

- *Cerebral hemorrhage* is usually caused by hypertension, or high blood pressure.

- *Subarachnoid hemorrhage* is a dangerous kind of stroke, the result of an *aneurysm*, a weakened blood vessel that has bulged like a balloon and can burst. The blood then flows into the subarachnoid space, a thin area between the skull and the brain. Sometimes this kind of stroke is caused by an abnormal connection between arteries and veins called an *arteriovenous malformation*.

Treatment of Hemorrhagic Stroke

Until recently, emergency surgical intervention was not very effective in saving the life of the victim of a hemorrhagic stroke, but the odds for survival have improved of late if the patient is treated quickly after onset. In other life-or-death situations, a *hemicraniectomy*—the surgical removal of a piece of skull to remove pressure on the brain caused by pooling blood—is performed. Another surgical method for relieving pressure on brain tissue is a *decompressive craniotomy,* which involves draining off blood through a small hole drilled into the skull.

Patients with subarachnoid hemorrhage typically undergo surgery when inflammation has gone down, usually within a few days after a stroke. If the aneurysm has ruptured, a clip is placed across the neck of the bulge to stop the bleeding. Because of the location of these aneurysms, surgery can be very difficult and may involve removing parts of the skull or lowering body temperature to reduce the bleeding.

If the aneurysm has not ruptured, surgery is controversial and may be unwarranted. All risks and options should be discussed with a specialist.

A promising new procedure, called a *transcatheter embolization for sealing off the aneurysm,* is now in clinical trial. A catheter is threaded through the artery involved and the aneurysm is sealed off from the artery wall. Already proved to be highly effective in treating both ruptured and unruptured aneurysms, this approach will be far less invasive and risky than the current procedures.

Nonsurgical Treatments for Hemorrhagic Stroke

After a subarachnoid stroke, there is a danger of spasm in the blood vessels near the rupture. *Calcium channel blockers* help relax those vessels. In severe cases the patient is put in a medically induced coma to ensure optimum healing conditions.

Loss of Function Caused by Stroke

The brain is amazingly complex, well ordered, and survival-oriented. Control of motor and sensory functions is delegated to specific regions. For example, an area behind the eye controls the sense of smell, and an area at the back of the brain is responsible for vision. The brain also is divided front to back into right and left hemispheres; the left hemisphere controls motor and sensory functions on the right side of the body, and the right hemisphere controls those functions on the left side. If a stroke has attacked the right hemisphere, it will affect the left side of the body and vice versa.

The hemispheres also divide responsibilities for the higher (cerebral) functions of the brain: the right hemisphere is in control of creativity, artistic abilities, and awareness, insight, and spatial orientation. The left hemisphere is responsible for language, both spoken and written, reasoning and logic, number skills, and scientific thought. In a general way, these functions can be reduced to two words: thinking (left brain) and feeling (right brain). These functions of the two hemispheres are reversed in left-hand-dominant people. The beautiful part is that an undamaged hemisphere can take over the responsibilities of a damaged hemisphere. That's what happened in Pasteur's case, in a time when nothing medically could be done to treat stroke.

Impairment caused by ischemic and hemorrhagic strokes is similar, depending on the severity of the stroke, the area of damage, and the extent to which one part of the brain is able to take over the functions of another. Keeping in mind that no two brains are alike, following is a description of the effects of the impairment that you may be observing in your loved one:

- Right-hand-dominant stroke patients suffer a loss of memory, attention span, spatial orientation, and emotional control. You may notice that the quiet and sober person you once knew is now impulsive, volatile, erratic, laughing one moment and crying the next for no apparent reason.

- If the left hemisphere of right-hand-dominant people has been attacked, patients will suffer communication problems, from difficulty with pronouncing words to a complete loss of speech. The ability to understand spoken and written language also is impaired. They also experience personality changes. The high-spirited, fun-loving, quick-witted person you knew may now be subdued and cautious, slow to respond, compulsive instead of impulsive, disorganized, and extremely frustrated by the loss of communication skills.

- The brains of left-hand-dominant people are bilateral, meaning that language and cognition are controlled by both hemispheres. As a consequence, their impairments will vary from those of right-hand-dominant people.

HELP A FAMILY SHARE THE RESPONSIBILITIES OF GUARDIANSHIP AND ENSURE CONTINUITY OF CARE

- Work out a schedule of shifts. If at all possible, make each person's shift at the same time each day. The hospital staff is also on a shift, and that way they can get to know you.

- Whoever is in charge of a shift should be the only person who communicates with the medical staff. It's the most efficient way for both family and staff to gather information and prevent confusion.

- Keep a notebook. Write down everything—tests, medication, whatever the medical staff reports. Whatever doesn't fit in the notebook can go in a big envelope that's kept in the hospital room, but record what it is in the notebook. This information also will come in handy when you need to deal with insurance companies or apply for government assistance. Being a vigilant record-keeper is not a reflection on the quality of care the patient is getting, but hospital staff do make mistakes. You're their backup.

- Patients who face the greatest challenges are those who have suffered damage in both hemispheres.

After a stroke, nearly all patients suffer to some degree from *dysphagia,* difficulty swallowing, and *dysarthria*, weakness of the muscles used in speech.

Being a Good Guardian

I'm sure all this information must have your head spinning. But you're not in school where you have to memorize it for tomorrow's test! This is real-life information for a different purpose: to refer to as the need arises. Not only will it help you understand what the doctors are telling you, but it also will help you understand what's happened to your loved one, who may not even know at this point what kinds of impairments have taken place.

4

Rebirth

———◆———

A T NINE O'CLOCK every morning, Monday through Friday, a
nurse helped me into my wheelchair and rolled me down
the corridor to rehab. Even though the therapies were hard
work, it felt good to be on a regular schedule again, with something important to do each day. I felt less like a patient and
more like the superachiever I had always been. Physical therapy came first, more challenging than any workout I had ever
done in a gym. In the beginning I had to rely completely on
Christine to move my flaccid limbs for me.

One exercise I remember well. With a wide belt secured
around my waist, I would get on my hands and knees and pick
up small colored cones that Christine had placed just outside
my reach. She would hold me up by the belt while I leaned forward, forcing me to put weight on my weak left side. Anyone
looking on would think that such a simple exercise was child's
play, but picking up those colored cones was so difficult that
my body trembled as tears rolled down my face.

When I had gained enough strength in my limbs, it was time
for me to learn how to crawl. I couldn't believe how difficult it

was—and still is! I had heard that babies must crawl before they can walk, but never having had children, I didn't know exactly why. Now I was finding out what an important role crawling plays in motor coordination. It creates a connection between the right and the left hemispheres of the brain that is necessary not only for walking but also for reading and hundreds of other important tasks. Since my stroke had affected both hemispheres, matters were even more complicated in my rehabilitation.

In those early days of starting over, there were times I would have given up if it hadn't been for the encouragement of all my therapists. They were extraordinary. Each one seemed personally motivated to help me reach my goal of being able to walk again. Their faith in me gave me the courage I needed to accomplish what seemed impossible at the time. Looking back on those early triumphs, it's clear to me that I was already moving mountains—I was beginning on my hands and knees.

I was excited to graduate to the parallel bars; it felt as though I was actually achieving the first steps toward my goal. As I held on to the bars, Christine would stand me up and move my paralyzed foot one step at a time as yet another therapist held on to me. They were careful not to cause any unnecessary discomfort, but it was evident that my desire to overcome my injury mattered more to me than the pain I suffered.

Next was speech therapy, which I always looked forward to because I wanted so badly to talk again. I prayed for that, even promising God that if I ever got my voice back, I would never stop talking about my recovery, inspiring other stroke survivors that even a total loss of speech could be overcome.

My speech therapist, Beth, taught me exercises for strengthening my cheek and tongue muscles, and I practiced them diligently in my room between sessions. One exercise required pulling out my tongue with my good hand while retracting it at the same time. The resistance helps to create strength. I didn't have gauze pads in my room to use for holding out my tongue, so I used my shirt instead. Naturally, this created a big wet spot—not pretty, but it worked. In time, I think my tongue could have pulled a car!

I also had to relearn how to identify numbers and pronounce the alphabet. Beth and I spent many hours with flash cards and puzzles to restore these cognitive skills. The relearning process was excruciatingly slow. I often thought about the million-dollar cases I used to work on for my clients. Just a few weeks before, I had been a whiz at numbers. Now I could hardly add or subtract.

Still, I was grateful that my memory and cognitive functions were returning. Not all the brain-injured patients in rehab were as lucky. I understood that each little gain was truly a gift, and I was grateful.

One morning Beth told me, "Valerie, it's time to give up your writing board so you can find your voice."

No way! I panicked at the thought. My writing board was my sole means of communication, and now Beth wanted to take it away! Though I was left-handed as a child, I had later learned to write with both hands. Thank God for my grade school teacher who had forced me to use my right hand.

"No!" I scratched out. I couldn't bear the thought of giving up my precious white erasable board! I'd only had it for a week. Previously, I had to write on every scrap piece of paper in sight, dependent on everyone to search for more paper.

"It will be tough at first," Beth said, reaching for my board, "but this is the only way you'll find your voice. And you only have to give it up when you're with me. I'll give it back to you after our sessions."

I acquiesced, lowering my head in humble acceptance as I surrendered my board to her. She was right—it was tough—and so maddening as I kept forgetting and would instinctively reach for it throughout our sessions.

Finally, one day a sound rose up in my throat and sprung out of my mouth. It was so weird. But I was thrilled. My vocal chords still worked! In the following days I made more sounds, all of them as strange as the first. This, however, was both difficult to do and disappointing for me. What was the use of making sounds if I still couldn't communicate?

"Valerie, this is hard work," Beth assured me. "It may not feel like you're making much progress yet, but you are. Your motivation is admirable. So many stroke survivors just give up. We have a saying around here: 'Some become better and some become bitter.'"

That stuck with me. Despite my frustration, I did not want to become bitter. Alone in my room, I practiced every exercise she gave me, and I even picked up a magazine someone had given me and tried reading aloud. I began with the cover. I knew the words, I understood their meaning, I heard them in my head, but when they came out, the sounds made no sense to me.

What on earth was that? When did I learn Russian? My attempt at speech was frightening, but I had to laugh.

I was beginning to discover that the more I was able to laugh at myself, the stronger I felt. My fighting spirit was reemerging and so was my sense of humor. The stroke became my opponent, and I found myself utilizing all my strength and courage to defeat it. Whenever the challenges would overwhelm me and bring me to my knees, I would personify my stroke and tell it, *"You haven't got me! No, sir! I've got you!"*

After a few intense weeks I sounded out my first word, the one I was required to say before I could be discharged: "Help!" It was followed by other words, each one a victory over my stroke. One particular word was accompanied by a fond memory.

When I was growing up, I raised dwarf rabbits in my backyard. I started out with one, then decided he needed a mate, and—well—you know the rest. Soon I had so many rabbits that I turned my backyard into my first business, delivering baskets of adorable baby bunnies to the local pet stores at Easter. My parents were supportive of my entrepreneurial spirit and grew equally fond of those furry little creatures. Though it may not seem so, "rabbit" is a difficult word to articulate, requiring many muscles of the mouth and tongue to work together, but I was determined. One day when Angie arrived, I looked up at her and proudly shouted, "Rabbit!"

"Val, you can talk!" she exclaimed.

"Rabbit," I agreed. "Rabbit!"

After that, I started learning a new word each day. Although "Valerie" is also difficult to articulate, I did manage to say my nickname, "Val." I was so proud. Back in my room, I phoned a friend who didn't know that I'd had a stroke, hoping she would recognize me.

"Hello," she said.

"V-v-a-a-a-l-l-l-l," I replied. I had sounded out each letter as clearly as I could and still sounded like a three-year-old, but I was so overjoyed when I heard my friend say, "Val, is that you?"

Tears filled my eyes. She knew it was me!

"Where are you?" she asked. That was a tough one to answer.

"H-h-h-osss-pittt-allll," I sounded out.

The call didn't last long, and after we hung up, she telephoned my mother to find out what I couldn't explain. A connection had been made, and that filled me with hope. I had taken another baby step in this new life—a rebirthing process—that had just begun.

My routine had changed dramatically from my life before the stroke, a time when I had been constantly on the go, meeting people morning, noon, and night. Now I had to find ways to break out of my isolation. Some days I'd sit in my wheelchair outside the gym and watch the new patients and their families go through orientation.

"In rehab we provide physical therapy, better known as PT,

occupational therapy or OT, and speech," the nurse told them. As I listened to her recite the standard speech, I sighed. I felt like an old-timer. Having been there a while, I knew the lingo: PT, which we patients often referred to as physical torture, was self-explanatory, and so was speech therapy. But OT, occupational therapy, was not. OT was my least favorite. It taught us how to use our fine motor skills and was the most frustrating of the three therapies.

Occupational therapy consists of repetitive tasks such as picking up pennies, putting pegs in a board, and identifying shapes with your eyes closed. What a pain! I'd rather be tortured in PT than go through this tedious process, but it was in OT that I learned to tie my shoes, cook, and make my bed with one hand—important skills to master as I strived for my independence again. My desire for self-sufficiency was so great that I willingly put up with the daily frustration of OT, giving it my all so I could relearn to do these things for myself.

Afternoons were free time. I spent the first week in my room, lost in my thoughts, until I nearly drove myself crazy. In desperation I joined the other patients in the gathering room, where we made crafts. Painting pottery and making hot plates had never been of any interest in my previous life, but you'd never have known it by the way I threw myself into these activities. In fact, I really was enjoying myself. My sister, however, was not buying it.

One day, after watching me making a hot plate, she couldn't take it any more and went looking for a nurse.

"This is too strange!" she told her. "This is not my sister. Valerie doesn't do crafts. She hates crafts! She would no more be caught making a hot plate than I would go fishing. Is this permanent? Or is she going to snap out of it?"

My poor sister; her nerves were shot. She didn't know whether to laugh or cry watching me happily doing arts and crafts in the gathering room. But she was right. I was changing. I was having fun being creative, just as I had been when I was a

child. Prior to the stroke, I had used my imagination for prag-
matic things such as making money and building businesses.
Now I was using it without any motivation at all, just the sheer
pleasure of creating things. And yes, this change *was* permanent. I'm still that way today. It became one of the hidden
treasures of my stroke survival.

The hospital offered other diversions, led by volunteers. One
day I checked the bulletin board where all these extra activities
were posted and noticed that haircuts were given on Tuesday
afternoons. Although I knew that a volunteer would never
come close to the professional skills of my hairdresser, my hair
looked so frightful that I couldn't stand it another day. I threw
caution to the wind and signed up. Tuesday couldn't come fast
enough for me.

The volunteer was nice but much older than any hairdresser
I'd ever seen. Naturally, I was a bit hesitant. But I was learning
how to surrender and go with the flow. I just kept telling
myself, *"It can't look any worse than it already does."*

Unfortunately, it did. Horrified, I sat in the chair as I witnessed my hair being cut from shoulder length to above my
ears, without any shape or style. I might as well have been bald.
I left the room wearing my baseball cap, humiliated. Hair
grows back, I told myself. I could survive this, too.

Once a week we had a group therapy session where we shared
stories about our strokes. When it was my turn, the therapist
explained that my voice was temporarily down for repairs.
Instead, I excelled at listening. Even though most of the patients
were thirty to forty years older than I was, we had all endured a
life-altering experience that had bonded us. One woman had
her stroke while riding her John Deere tractor, mowing her
property. Just about every time I saw her, she asked me, "When
you get out of here, will you go mow my yard?" Another elderly woman had lain on her floor for three days, just two feet
from her phone, until her housekeeper found her.

As I listened to these other patients tell their stories, I felt less alone. It's impossible for people to understand what it's like to suffer a brain injury unless it's happened to them. I began to feel safe with my fellow patients and grew to care deeply about them. I had a special concern for the prognosis of some of the older ones. The survival statistics were not in their favor.

My heart also went out to a teenage girl who'd been severely injured and lost an eye in a terrible car accident. She was lucky to be alive, but I knew sometimes she didn't feel that way. Every day during my free time I'd wheel myself down to her room, and if she was awake and up for company she would wave and gesture that I could come in. Neither of us could talk, but somehow we were able to communicate. We were the youngest patients in the unit and had an unspoken bond. Although I yearned to go home, that day became bittersweet in my mind. I knew it would be hard to leave these new friends.

My discharge date was still up in the air because my prognosis remained uncertain. In the meantime, I was determined to take control of my own outcome regardless of what any doctor or pamphlet might say. In fact, I threw away the *Stroke Care* manual they gave me. I didn't want to fill my head with ideas and pictures of what might lie ahead of me. I wanted to create my own outcome. Of course, my caregivers had to be aware of the effects of stroke to be prepared to care for me properly, but I strongly believe that what we fear *will* come upon us. I wanted to focus on how I could make myself better as quickly as possible.

A family friend, Eloise, was a reflexologist. She came to the hospital several times a week to give me foot massages. She taught me that rubbing the bottom of your big toes stimulates the brain and blood flow. These sessions helped me so much that I also continued treatment with a reflexologist during my recovery at home.

Each Friday I attended a meeting with all my doctors and

therapists to discuss my progress. Family members also were invited, but they weren't available at that time, so Eloise attended in their absence. These meetings were semiformal, with the staff taking turns to describe my progress, but it always felt like they were grading me—and they were. At the end of the meeting they asked me if I had anything I would like to add. Each time I would nod my head, take out my board, and write the word "Home."

I was so homesick that my sisters decided to cheer me up by decorating my room. My younger sister, Michelle, brought me a wind chime and hung it from the overhead rail of my bed. She also brought a little machine that filled the room with the pleasant sound of crickets at night and the peaceful lapping of ocean surf during the day. Doctors passing by would tell me, "I'm coming back to your room to relax!" A framed photograph of my cat, Alex, sat on my dresser. Flowers and get-well cards covered every shelf and available floor space. At one point I ran out of room and started giving the flowers to other patients.

No matter what people did for me to make my stay more comfortable, or how hard I worked during the day, nothing seemed to help make the time pass faster. The hours especially dragged slowest at night. Each day I assured myself that I was another day closer to going home. Each night I thanked God for helping me make it through another day and asked for the strength and courage to make it through the next.

On the Fourth of July I had to try extra hard to cheer myself up, but it was too sad. Tears streamed down my face as I watched the downtown fireworks from a hospital window, reminiscing about the good times I'd had celebrating in past years, surrounded by friends. Returning to my room, I phoned a few friends. Not all of them recognized my garbled attempt at saying my name. Some of them hung up, but just hearing their voices made me feel like I was still in the same world, only on another side of it.

The physical distance from my parents during this time was also very difficult. Sadly, Mom and I were unable to resolve our differences that continued to surface and cause stress to my heightened nerves. Dad, who also stayed away, struggled with not being able to cope with seeing me in this condition. Though I know they loved me dearly, I learned something valuable from both of them. I learned that no matter how painful it may be to see someone who is suffering, and no matter what your differences may be, it is so important to be present, especially with loved ones. It is not about words or gifts or even sympathy. They simply need us to be near.

My big sister, Angie, really was my saving grace. Busy as she was with her own family hundreds of miles away in Florida's panhandle, she came to the hospital as often as she could, faithful and reliable. I knew that no matter what happened, she would be there for me. I'll never forget how I would wait by my hospital window in the afternoons, looking for her to pull up to the curb in her silver minivan and take me out for a couple of hours. Sometimes we would just ride down Park Avenue, a stylish street of shops, cafés, and restaurants, or simply ride by my house in Winter Park. It didn't matter where we went; I was just happy to get out.

Near the end of my hospital stay, I was given a catalog to pick out my wheelchair. They came in all kinds of designs and colors. As I turned the pages, my anger grew. I did not intend to live my life in a wheelchair! I would not accept that as an option! I closed the catalog and slung it out into the hallway as hard as I could throw. Thunk! It smacked against the wall across from my open door.

The nurses were very understanding about my anger and, thank God, they were also tolerant of my mischievousness. Single-handedly, I kept the staff on their toes. I was always trying to escape from the rehab wing. Fortunately, my room was at the far end of a hallway that was closed off by double automated doors that led to the main lobby and cafeteria. Each day after lunch I would sit in my wheelchair in the doorway of my room and watch the doctors and nurses enter and exit through those doors, memorizing when their shifts changed. I discovered that during the lunch hours they would leave the doors open for about ten minutes. The sounds of shuffling feet and the aroma of fresh-baked chocolate chip cookies filled the hallways just beyond the doors.

I longed for one of those cookies! My scheme was to make a getaway into the cafeteria during that ten-minute window while the doors were open. The day finally came when I could make my move. I worked my wheelchair with my good leg, edged out of my room into the hallway, and waited. Sure enough, like clockwork, the shift returning from lunch had left the doors open. I looked down the hall. The coast was clear!

Off I rolled. I made it through the doors without being seen, and then casually wheeled myself down the hall. I was doing fine until I came to an area where the floor sloped down. What a bizarre design for a hospital, I thought. By keeping my good foot against the floor to control the speed of my wheelchair, I managed to ease my way safely down the slope. At the bottom was the cafeteria. I was in ecstasy! What a woman won't do for chocolate!

The self-service counter was low enough for my wheelchair, so I managed to get a few cookies and a pint of milk. Going through the checkout line, I presented my patient ID. Since patients didn't need to pay, the clerk waved me through and I proceeded to a nearby table to slowly enjoy my cookies and milk. Just being surrounded by real food was heavenly. My senses were going crazy. I could smell pizza, coffee, and the wonderful aroma of those fresh-baked cookies.

After nearly an hour had passed, the nurses discovered that I was missing from my room, and the search began. Much to my dismay, it wasn't long before I heard my name being called, and I was found. After listening to a lecture, I realized that my escape was not the best decision I could have made. Many things could have happened to me, like falling down or injuring myself, but that had never entered my mind.

When I returned to PT the next morning, my little escapade was headline news among the therapists. Somehow I remained in good standing with the staff, even though they did seem to check my room more frequently.

One day Angie hung a large bow on my door and said I was being crowned a "star patient." Ha! Star pain was probably more like it! I was pretty sure this was my sister's psychology at work, hoping I would now be required to behave in a manner that would live up to my star image.

As the weeks of rigorous therapy continued, I could feel myself growing stronger, both mentally and physically. At last the day came that I had been impatiently looking forward to for so long. The authorization came through for my discharge the following Monday, with a home health care nurse and a continued outpatient rehab program. I was going *home*!

One of my last visitors brought me even more joy. Milton was a lifelong friend. We had known each other since first grade and had kept in touch since then. Now he stood next to my wheelchair, holding out flowers. Looking at his warm smile, unable to speak, I could only cry.

"Valerie, when you get out of here, I'll take you to my doctor," he told me. "I know he can help you. You can beat this!"

I believed him. And good friend that he had always been, he kept his promise.

After the longest weekend of my life, Monday morning arrived. I sat on my bed, packed and fully dressed, waiting for Angie. Upon her arrival, she collected my discharge orders and papers. If you have ever stayed in a hospital, you know that this can take forever. While I was waiting, I sprayed my room with an entire can of pink Silly String that my sister Michelle had given to me. I'm sure she didn't expect me to use it indoors, but it helped express my joy.

I also stopped by every room to say good-bye to the friends I had made during my long stay. I cried as I hugged each person, knowing that I might not ever see them again. I had become so close to my fellow stroke survivors; the outstanding, dedicated nurses who cared for me; and the amazing therapists who pushed me beyond what I ever imagined I could do.

Before we left, Angie and I made one last stop, at the gift shop, where I purchased something for each of the nurses and staff who had cared for me. Because I couldn't express my gratitude verbally, I hoped my gifts would help them understand how much they meant to me. They had helped me begin the process of reclaiming my life. Though filled with joy at the anticipation of my homecoming, deep within I knew I'd need to find a way to continue on my own.

I didn't know, then, the mountains that still lay ahead.

Exciting "New" Findings

*What's happening now is the rediscovery of old ideas
made modern with new technology.*

—James F. Toole, M.D., president of the
International Stroke Society

SO MANY CHANGES have recently taken place that the first ten years of the twenty-first century are already being called the "decade of the brain." Until the advent of highly sophisticated imaging tools, neurological research was limited to the study of dead brains, which is like trying to find out how a complex machine operates without the motor running, or by observing the behavior of patients with damaged brains. Now a whole new world of exploration in the workings of a living brain has researchers excited about the future. That kind of news makes headlines, but this knowledge is not "news" so much as a confirmation in the laboratory of what neurologists have been observing all along.

As late as the mid-1990s, the orthodox opinion in stroke medicine was that loss of function due to the death of nerve cells was permanent because the brain didn't replace them. This pessimistic conclusion may account for the lack of interest in or treatment for stroke recovery. When a respected neuroscientist published a study showing how exercise resulted in the growth of brain cells in mice, the concept of "neurogenesis" captured the attention of the neuroscientific community. Then, when the same results were replicated for the first time in a human brain, neurologists started talking about an "explosion of knowledge" in their field.

Many neurologists who have treated stroke patients for years have never doubted that the brain can recover. In the 1890s a physician received the Nobel Prize for putting together the two ends of a severed spinal cord and making it grow. Do these new studies really show the birth of new neurons, or is exercise revitalizing neurons that have been there all along but never got used before? Could it be that these reactivated neurons are creating new pathways, or that more of them are connecting with one another?

And do these arguments really matter to the stroke patients who want to recover, or to the therapists who treat them? I don't know, but the recent discoveries already are having an effect on the stroke rehabilitation community. They are rethinking long-held assumptions about the recoverable brain, especially that patients could not recover beyond six months after a stroke. During training, therapists were told to stop seeing patients after that time because nothing more would change in motor or language skills. Any improvements after six months were the result of patients' willingness to adjust to their condition and learn ways of adapting to it. Even when therapists were surprised to see real recovery in cognitive and motor skills, they had no statistics to back it up.

What the recent studies *do* provide is statistical proof of the connection between exercise and the brain, which many rehabilitation professionals have known all along through observation. Now physical therapists know that when they exercise the arms, legs, and even the chin of a stroke survivor, they're assisting the brain in finding new ways to reconnect with these body parts. When speech therapists urge family members to keep a conversation going with a patient, no matter how fruitless their efforts may seem, they can assure loved ones that this effort assists in the recovery of a patient's cognitive abilities. Because of these recent breakthroughs in knowledge about the recoverable brain, no longer are family members and friends helpless onlookers in the aftermath of a stroke. Now they have a crucial role to play in the recovery process.

How Family and Friends Can Help

Imagine going to sleep one night and waking up in a foreign country. Your mental faculties are the same, but you can't understand the language or be understood by others. That's what it's like for many survivors of a massive stroke—only worse. It's their own country they wake up in, and they're supposed to know the language, but suddenly they don't. That's what aphasia feels like, but family members need to understand that aphasia impairs language and speech more than it impairs thinking. Imagine the frustration! Here are some guidelines for caregivers that will help them find a new way to communicate with their loved ones.

- Consult with the hospital's speech therapist, whose expertise is establishing patients' levels of understanding and communication as soon as they are conscious. These therapists convey that information to the nurses. You need it, too.

- Early on, you may be saying all the right things, but the patients are not taking it in. Much more important than what you're saying is how you're saying it. Are you holding their hand? What's the tone of your voice? However you can, connect with them in a loving way. More than anything you can say, that's what comforts them.

- If they are not able to communicate verbally but are able to comprehend, you can ask questions that can be answered with a yes-no response, indicated by a gesture, such as an eye blink or a finger tap.

- Communicate with them visually what they're missing auditorially, and convey this to family and friends so the time they spend with the patient is more fruitful. For example, if you want to talk about their grandchildren, bring along their pictures. Wherever possible, give visual cues. If you're going to the cafeteria, make a gesture that conveys your message. Visual cues make patients feel more secure, because they can anticipate what's going to happen.

- Expect that if they do get their voice back, their speech will be distorted. Try not to look dismayed. Instead, convey gratitude that your loved one's vocal powers have been restored.

- Talk to them calmly. Don't raise your voice. One of the most difficult aspects of stroke recovery is losing one's adult standing. People start talking loudly and condescendingly, as if the patient were deaf or mentally impaired, or a child. Even worse, people talk about them instead of to them.

- Be vigilant by insisting that visitors treat the patient with respect. They're at the whim of whoever walks in and tries to figure out what they need. They can't even make a simple request such as "Can you get me my robe?" Patients feel that they've already lost so much of what they once took for granted. Don't allow their dignity to be taken away from them, too.

- As your loved one's understanding improves, try not to throw a lot of information at them at once. Some people come in and talk a blue streak while the patient sits by, not able to follow the conversation and feeling like he or she is on the outside, looking in.

- Go to my Web site at www.thefirewithin.com, click on "Caregivers," and print out the forty-two-page book *Stroke Caregivers Handbook*, which is based on the experiences of many caregivers to stroke survivors. The author, Joyce Dreslin, has given permission to Stroke Awareness for Everyone (SAFE) to distribute the book for free through the Internet. The information she provides about the responsibilities of caregivers and the special needs of survivors poststroke is much more thorough than I can pro-

WHAT CAREGIVERS NEED RIGHT NOW

A stroke doesn't affect just the patient; it also affects the entire family. Everyone is going through a grieving process. They have truly lost the person they had before and are now facing a new way of existing. At the same time, they must comfort and care for the one who has lost the most— this helpless, afraid, angry, confused, depressed, utterly changed person they once knew—when their own life, and most likely their future plans, have been turned upside down. If there was ever a time to learn how to say "Yes!" when people ask "How may I help you?," it's now.

Many people are much more comfortable giving than receiving, or are so independent or unwilling to burden others that they might have trouble delegating responsibilities or even thinking of things that can be done by others. Is there a dog that needs to be walked? Are cell phones prohibited and you've run out of quarters for the pay phone? Friends and relatives will welcome specific requests, knowing they are being truly helpful. Here are some other ways to care for yourself.

- *Continuity.* On your hours off, try to maintain your normal life as much as possible: going to the gym, meeting friends, whatever makes you feel connected with the outside world.

- *A good night's sleep.* If you have trouble sleeping, have a physician prescribe a sleep aid. If you are reluctant to rely on medication or are worried about getting addicted, sleep aids are now available that aren't habit-forming. If you lie awake at night worrying, remind yourself that you're in a crisis. Times like this are what sleep aids are for, and a good night's sleep will make all the difference in your ability to cope with whatever tomorrow will bring.

- *Diversion.* Buy some good books, nothing that requires a lot of concentration, just entertaining page-turners that can give you some diversion while you're on bedside duty.

- *Nutrition.* Don't forget to eat. People in shock often lose their appetite. If that's the case for you, make sure that what you do manage to eat is not a candy bar. You need real nourishment.

- *Cooperation.* Make a list of all the responsibilities you can let go, whatever can be put off for now. When you call people to explain what's happened, they also may want to help. Remember: never decline. At the very least they can make phone calls for you. Nothing is more debilitating than telling people the story of the crisis over and over again, reliving it every time you hear the same shocked response. Delegate, delegate.

- *Self-comfort.* Acknowledge that you're grieving. You have lost someone. The patient is no longer the person you knew. Expect to feel anger, denial, depression, bargaining—all the well-known phases of the grieving process. It's natural, and it's your right to go through it.

- *Support.* Seek an emotional outlet from a therapist, support group, clergy, social worker, or someone close you can trust. It's very stressful being cheerful, understanding, and full of hope in front of the patient when you feel like falling apart. If you don't find an appropriate place to unload these feelings, you're not taking care of yourself!

vide in this book—compassionate and even humorous as well as practical. This group has been there and done that, and their collective wisdom may be just what you need.

You Made the Cut!

The best approach for everyone—patient, family, and friends— is one that Terese, my speech pathologist, calls hopeful reality. It's the philosophy that got me through that painful poststroke period.

I'm not taking hope away, but I tell my patients, "Let's just deal with what you need to do today and then we'll hope for something else tomorrow. Do you know how few people survive what you've gone through? You made the big cut! You can't give up now. There must be a plan for you. We just need to figure out what it is."

5

On My Own

———◆———

WHEN ANGIE WHEELED ME down the long brick walkway
that led to my house, I felt like a wounded soldier
returning home from a war. For a month and two days I had
battled for my life, and now I was a civilian again, free to enjoy
the comfort of an everyday routine at home. I could eat what I
wanted, when I wanted, and sleep in my own luxurious bedroom. No more rattling carts, no more predawn interruptions,
no more needles stuck in me around the clock! How I had
longed for the restoration of my freedom and independence.
Had I known, however, what challenges awaited me, I might
have balked. But at the time I was clueless and simply enjoyed
the moment.

Angie rolled me up the wheelchair ramp that my friend Tom
had built over the stairs to my front porch and unlocked the
front door to my beautifully remodeled 1800s Key West–style,
two-story house. I drank in the sight of my elegant surroundings where everything had meaning. My lungs filled with the
familiar scents of polished mahogany furniture, candles, and
wood floors. The smell of hospital disinfectants was behind me.

Where was Alex? He usually greeted me at my front door. Beyond the tall columns that framed the formal dining room, I saw his little face peering at me from the den. Out of habit I tried to call him, but I couldn't say his name. Instead of jumping into my lap and giving me his usual greeting, he turned tail and ran. Cats have a very clear way of letting you know when their feelings have been hurt, and my prolonged absence had clearly caused my feline friend much misery. Though disappointed, I felt sure that in time my faithful companion would forgive me.

Angie stayed with me for a few days, but then she had to return to her family. Although I was grateful she could stay, I was a little insecure about being alone. Having always been independent, I was confident that I could manage with some part-time help. Angie had arranged for a nurse from a local service to come every morning to bathe and dress me and to return every evening to help me get ready for bed. I could also depend on my housekeeper, Maxine, who came once a week.

I was so happy to be home that I hadn't given any thought to the hardships I would face alone. My house was not suited for a wheelchair or physical challenges. It was designed with a steep stairway to the second floor, with only one banister, on the left side. This meant that for me to use the staircase, I had to hold on to the left banister with my right hand. One false move and I was a goner. Of course, my physical therapist had strongly advised me to avoid stairs, but both my office and my beautiful bedroom were on the second floor. I just loved the feeling of being upstairs. Looking out my bedroom window at all the surrounding trees made me feel as though I were in a tree house. As a child, I had lived across the street from a heavily wooded piece of property, where my friends and I enjoyed building and playing in our tree forts high above the ground. Being upstairs reminded me of those happy times.

Determined to master those stairs, I would wheel my chair over to the stairs and slide myself onto the first step, get into a standing position, and with my strong right arm pull myself up one step at a time, dragging my left leg behind me like a heavy rag doll. Each week, Maxine would scrub the marks off the wood floors and stairs that were made by my lagging left foot. She was always sure to tell me how well I was doing and encouraged me to keep up the hard work.

Although I was increasingly lonely at night, I wasn't afraid. But that all changed the first night I awoke unable to breathe and choking on saliva that I had aspirated into my windpipe. The stroke had paralyzed my soft palate, which makes swallowing difficult. When it happened in the hospital, the nurses had come running. At home, alone, I'd choke and gag for thirty minutes sometimes before I was able to breathe normally again. I knew that aspiration is one of the major hazards a patient faces poststroke. Though I was panic-stricken, I was determined to remain independent.

Waking up to use the bathroom at night was another major challenge, especially when I didn't have my cane nearby. Fortunately, I had relearned how to crawl. I'd slide off the bed and crawl to the door, then pull myself up by grabbing the doorknob. As I leaned against the wall for support, I made my way down the long hallway to the bathroom. Sometimes I just couldn't make it in time and I'd wet myself. Then I'd be up for the next half hour, struggling to change into dry clothes and get back into bed.

During times like this I felt so abandoned. It was becoming increasingly apparent that I needed help badly. Often I would cry myself back to sleep. At other times I was wide awake with anger. *Why did this have to happen to me? Why do I have to go through this all by myself?*

I learned to survive, a day at a time. It helped having a nurse check on me each morning and evening. She was strong and nurturing, and she gave me the emotional support I needed nearly as much as the physical help. I wasn't always easy to care for, as I had refused most of the hospital's home health-care products that had been recommended, such as the shower chair. *Heck, no!* I shuddered at the very idea of sitting in my elegant black tub in a pathetic white plastic chair. Fortunately, my nurse could assist me into and out of the tub.

Thank God for my faithful friends who came by to visit and bring me food. I was grateful for their support and genuine kindness. At the same time, I was terribly hurt by a number of people I had once considered friends who never came by or even telephoned. It wasn't until years later, while working through my emotional trauma, that I was able to forgive them. In hindsight it's easy to see how fearful they must have been and how helpless they must have felt. But their absence caused me deep pain that I ultimately needed to forgive them for.

Before the stroke, my days had been frantically full. Now the big event of my week was going to rehab three days each week in addition to my constant doctor visits. On the rehab mornings, a small red and white bus picked me up at my door and, along with several others on board, took me to therapy sessions. The bus was a municipal public service provided to those who qualified. It cost only a dollar, which fascinated me. I never knew anything could still cost only a dollar. I would get so excited to see that bus pull up to my house. I'd be dressed in my sweats, waiting and raring to go.

Every day was a step closer to recovery. I might have fallen, but I was climbing my way back up! Though these sessions were extremely helpful, they exhausted me physically and overloaded me mentally. Getting my body to move was diffi-cult, but the hardest part was exercising my brain simultane-ously, as I urged it to send signals to my muscles again.

Aside from my therapy sessions, most of my time was spent trying to do simple tasks around my house. Just to be able to

turn the hose on and off to water my flowers was a challenge.
First I had to figure out how I was going to step down off the
wood deck in my backyard to reach the hose. Then, once I was
down there, how would I get back up? Everything required
great thought and precision. Sometimes I would spend so long
planning my moves that I would become hungry or tired, or it
would become too dark outside before I could accomplish my
goal.

Day after day I sat on my front porch swing with Alex
curled up next to me, waiting for the mailman or hoping to see
a familiar face. I was never a big fan of television, and my comprehension was too limited to read a book; I'd get frustrated
just trying to read through one page. I reminisced about the
time when I was eleven years old and my father hired a classical guitar instructor to teach me. In no time at all I advanced to
playing the twelve-string. My teacher observed that I had an
incredible ability to play by ear. Now, in my solitude, with my
mute twelve-string guitar staring at me, I longed to be able to
play once again.

Never in my life could I remember being lonely. I had never
known what it was to be bored. Now they were my constant
companions—loneliness and boredom. At times I felt as
though loneliness was a presence—a hovering demon, engulf-
ing me, making me feel rejected and useless. Many nights I lay
awake wondering why God had kept me alive. Why hadn't He
just let me die? In all honesty, taking my life had entered my
mind. Though I knew I would be greatly missed by my family
and friends, I hoped that they would understand. This person I
had become just wasn't me. I felt like a burden to my loved
ones, an unbearable thought for someone like me who champi-
oned self-sufficiency.

Yet whenever I was haunted by these thoughts, I heard an
inner voice telling me not to give up. I knew in my heart that I
was alive for a reason, that my journey was not complete. I
became aware that my stroke was to be a defining moment in

my life. It was almost as if I had been preparing for it all my life. In hindsight, I could see the signs. Prior to my stroke, when I'd work out, I felt as though I was training for something besides having a good figure. Doing leg lunges down a long hall with weights till I fell over from exhaustion, and arm curls till my biceps popped, I realized that I had pushed myself to great strength. I was grateful for that hard work as I now pulled the dead weight of my left leg up the stairs by the singular strength of my right arm.

It also occurred to me that I owed a debt of gratitude to my first-grade teacher. She had played an important role in my destiny when she insisted that I learn to write using my right hand.

"No one else in the class writes with their left hand," she had complained to me.

She was very strict. Knowing that I didn't want to appear different from the other kids or go against her wishes, I forced myself to switch to writing with my nondominant right hand. Had that teacher not insisted, I wouldn't have been able to communicate immediately after the stroke, and perhaps not for a very long and arduous time thereafter. I'd watched many of my fellow stroke survivors struggle to write with their nondominant hand. It would have been yet another difficult obstacle to overcome. I now saw my teacher's insistence as a gift.

It also was a gift that I was never a big eater. Food was simply fuel to me, and I didn't need much. Now my meals consisted of anything that was readily available, and that didn't bother me. Most important to me was that it was accessible. Angie had stocked my kitchen with lots of easy-to-open foods such as yogurt, fruit mix, and banana pudding—my favorite— and I quickly discovered all the things that are extremely difficult to do one-handed: peel a banana, open a can, or cut food. When my survivor instincts kicked in, I learned to use my teeth to assist me. Yet some things were beyond my ingenuity, such as opening a bag of potato chips or reaching for an item in the freezer. I had to wait to accomplish such tasks, humbled and frustrated at my limitations, until my nurse arrived.

"You should go out to lunch or dinner sometime," said my nurse. I stared at her in bewilderment as if to say, "Yeah, right!" I was embarrassed to be seen in public and fearful that I might encounter someone I knew. Not only did I look dreadful, I couldn't even talk.

Uncannily, the very next day my friend Tom came by and offered to take me out to lunch on a regular basis. *Oh, dear, now what?* I was torn. My thoughts raced.

I do want to go out! I want to ride in the car and hear the engine roar and the wind blow through my hair. I want to sit in traffic and hear a horn blow. But look at me. I can't be seen like this. I can't always wear a baseball cap and dark sunglasses. I walk like Bambi, and if I utter a sound, people will stare. And how am I supposed to keep from drooling when half my mouth is numb—paralyzed?

Putting all those fearful thoughts aside, I answered with a big, bright smile. "Yes, I'll go!"

We went to restaurants where I was least likely to run into people I knew. We frequented Holiday House, where my father had taken my family on Sundays after church when my sisters and I were children. Dad would ask for a table near the large window that overlooked the racetrack so we could watch the horses practice during our meal. The restaurant had lost its former grandeur, but it was still famous for serving extraordinary desserts. Banana cake was my favorite. I was comfortable going there because many customers were elderly and, in their midst, my disability wasn't as obvious. My cane was just one of many already there.

When Tom wasn't available to take me out, I had other resources. I learned to fax delivery requests to Pizza Hut. This girl was not going to starve!

Another gift from the past was Alex, who now played an important role in my new life. He'd been with me for seven years, since he was a kitten. Alex walked on a leash and loved riding in my car down Park Avenue wearing his leopard scarf. He even flew with me when I traveled. We had always been close, but now he was more than my companion; he also was my guardian. Before my stroke he had enjoyed his time alone, napping on the deck for hours in the shade. Now he never left my side. Every night he would run to the top of the stairs and wait for me as I pulled myself up, one slow step at a time. I felt as if he was cheering me on. Once I reached the top of the staircase, he would run to my bedroom and wait for me on my bed, where he would stay through the night until my nurse arrived in the morning. Alex was so attentive that I felt as if he had become an angel in disguise who watched over and protected me.

There were even times when I felt like we could read each other's thoughts. One early evening while sitting in my den I heard Alex growling as he stared out the French doors that lined the back of my house. For a cat, especially Alex, that was very odd. I had heard him hiss maybe a dozen times in his life. But growl? Never. He was obviously scared, and now so was I. What could be outside those doors? Alex's eyes grew wider.

When I looked out the door, I saw nothing at first.

"Alex, what do you see out there?" He continued to growl. Obviously it was still out there; I just couldn't see who or what it was. Then, in the lower left side of the door, I saw it. A little furry bandit wearing a mask.

"Oh, Alex, it's only a raccoon." I was relieved.

I reached for the door and tossed an Oreo cookie to the little fellow. I had never seen a raccoon up close. I watched as he held the cookie in his front paws and devoured it. He was adorable.

The next night, as I sat in my den, Alex began to growl again. Our little visitor was back, but this time he had brought his entire family—brothers, sisters, aunts, uncles, and cousins. Big and small, they covered every inch of the deck. It was like

Alfred Hitchcock's movie *The Birds,* except with raccoons.

Now what? We were outnumbered—twenty to two. As I reached for the bag of cookies, Alex reared up and looked at me. *"Do not open that door!"* I felt he was saying.

I hesitated. *Okay, maybe he's right.* It was a bit spooky. They did look like gremlins with a plan, especially the big ones.

My neighborhood was safe, as is most of Winter Park, and that safety is taken very seriously. So when a letter arrived from our local neighborhood association warning us about a rabid raccoon on the loose, I was bewildered. In the poststroke, diminished functioning of my brain, I was completely oblivious to what this meant. I tilted my head, puzzled at the word "rabid." Perhaps they had misspelled the word "rabbit." My scrambled brain concluded that a rabbit and a raccoon had mated.

Big deal! I promptly tossed the flyer in the garbage, not realizing at the time that my Alex had become my "watch" cat and had kept me safe.

At times I was like an innocent little child, living alone, not sure of what to do or expect. My guard was down, my protective instincts had been injured, and I had become very innocent. Worst of all, I didn't realize it.

The weeks passed, and my feelings of isolation grew. I decided to ask a friend to arrange for a limousine to pick me up and take me out for the evening. If I had learned one thing from my stroke, it was that life is short and you'd better enjoy it while you can. I was determined to make the best of it. When John, the limo driver, arrived, I handed him a written explanation of my disability and a list of places where I wanted to go. He drove me down Park Avenue, then to one of my favorite cafés to buy ice cream. I stayed in the limo as he went inside to fill my order. We drove around most of the evening, riding past familiar places that brought back such fond memories. It was nine o'clock when the limo returned to my house. John opened the car door and helped me out. I used my cane, and he politely held my left arm as we made our way up the brick walkway to the house. The ride had been relaxing and had enabled me to forget my troubles for a while.

Long after I had gone to bed that night, I was awakened by the phone ringing. It was two o'clock in the morning. I picked up the receiver and listened.

"Hi, Valerie," said a slightly familiar male voice. "This is John, your limo driver. I'm coming over to visit you. I'll be there in a few minutes."

Unable to respond, I quickly hung up the receiver and dialed 911, frightened out of my wits. No one visits at that hour, especially not your limo driver. As soon as the operator answered, I barely got out in a faint voice: "Help!"

Police officers arrived shortly after my call and walked throughout my property. They did not see anyone and left their card, insisting that I call if this man phoned me again. Fortunately, I didn't hear from him again, nor did I pursue any other limo reservations for a while. It was distressing and disheartening to realize that there really are people in this world who prey on those who are disabled.

Day after day, I'd sit on my front porch swing, waiting for the mailman or hoping for a visitor to come by. One morning, to my surprise, a truck pulled up in the driveway. It was Milton! He had come to fulfill his promise to help me.

"Val, I'm here to take you to a special doctor I know," he said.

Of all my friends, I'd known Milton the longest. We met in first grade. He was a cute boy with curly hair. Our mothers met at our class Christmas party, and as they grew to be best friends, so did we.

He put my wheelchair into his truck and we drove off. Arriving at a large office building, Milton carefully pushed me in my wheelchair up the ramp and into the elevator.

While sitting in the doctor's waiting room, I looked over

some brochures that outlined the alternative procedures in which the doctor specialized. Some of them I recognized, but I had no idea what stem cell injections or hyperbaric oxygen treatments were. When I was growing up, my mother was very health-conscious. We had a traditional family physician, but Mom always sought holistic treatments to complement our care. Having this background as a child, I learned to be open but cautious. Not all care—traditional or holistic—is good care. Also, I knew that in my current condition, my choices were limited. I refused to stay this way. I desperately needed help, and I was trusting that I had found it.

Moments later, a nurse came out and said we could see the doctor. Winding down a long hallway, past many rooms, we came to a large office at the end of the hall.

The walls of the doctor's office were covered with framed degrees in traditional medicine, but the office was eccentrically decorated with a red sofa and animal skins. Sitting behind a large glass desk, peering into a microscope, was a man wearing a white lab coat and cowboy boots. *Hmmm . . . different.* He welcomed us and asked how he could help. Milton spoke for me, explaining my condition. When the doctor learned of the severity of my stroke, he looked at me with compassion, then described his program and how it could help me. I was surprised to hear that it required leaving the country for a month and going to an offshore medical facility he owned and operated in the Dominican Republic.

The doctor showed me a number of magazine articles endorsing his work. I was impressed. His program had been noted for its amazing results with patients who had a stroke or another severe injury. He also gave us the name of a trial lawyer and former patient who lived in a nearby city. I wrote a note to the doctor, asking him if I could hear from this patient about his experience, and the doctor immediately dialed his number. The former patient's wife answered the phone and said she would be glad to talk to me, as her husband wasn't home. She described how he had been so badly injured and how he had been at the point of suicide. She then told me how his condition had dramatically improved after being treated at the doctor's clinic. The best news she gave me was that her husband wasn't home because he was busy working on a trial. After hearing her testimony, together with the doctor's many credentials and other endorsements, I was convinced of his credibility. For the first time since my stroke I was filled with hope.

Unfortunately, the treatment was not covered by insurance, and the cost was more than I could afford or anyone in my family could manage at the time. Discouraged, I didn't know how I could have this treatment without the necessary funds. In addition, since the best results were achieved as soon after an injury as possible, time was of the essence.

A few days passed, and my friends Lori and Helen, business and golfing buddies, heard of my need. Helen owned an Allstate Insurance agency in Winter Park, and Lori was a broker with a large insurance firm. They went into action at once and organized a golf tournament and auction to raise funds for my treatment, gathering donations from celebrities and local businesses, many of whom had once been clients of my firm and were eager to help.

More than a hundred people came to the event, including a local sports celebrity who signed autographs. Angie also attended and was given a large hat donated by a local designer. It was an amazing concoction of rhinestones and bows. I'm surprised it didn't play music! With her long blond hair, she wore it well.

Words will never be able to express the amount of love and support I felt that day and how my spirits were lifted. Nearly all the money I needed for the treatment was raised.

A trust was formed and plane reservations were made. I had a week to get any last-minute things in order. I was leaving the country to undergo live stem cell treatments. Unsure of what to expect, I put all my fears aside and placed my trust in God to take care of me.

My good friend and veterinarian Dr. Sandy Fink offered to care for Alex while I was away. Pat Peters, my massage therapist, agreed to accompany me through my first week of treatment. Pat was someone I enjoyed being around. She was a kind, older woman whom I trusted. Having her companionship was a great comfort to me.

Preparing for the trip, I was anxious and scared. I was uncertain how my body would respond to the treatment or how I would manage in unfamiliar surroundings as well as in a foreign country.

Dr. Fink came to my house to pick up Alex. With tears streaming down my face, I held my dear pet tightly and kissed him good-bye. My throat burned from the pain of not knowing if it was the last time I would see him. My only comfort was knowing that he would be in good hands.

My nurse helped pack my suitcase with the barest of necessities. Workout attire was about the only clothing I could wear because I couldn't yet manage zippers or buttons. This time my absence was planned, and a photograph of Alex was among the few mementos I packed to remind me of home.

I just didn't know whether I would ever return.

Homecoming and the Caregiver

A S I LOOK BACK on my experiences following my stroke, I realize how many risks I took that shouldn't ever have been made. I had no idea how vulnerable I was, given my state of mind. I was just so glad to be home, I wasn't aware of my cognitive shortcomings and challenges in addition to my physical impairments. That's a potentially dangerous situation for anyone to be in, and you can't always count on luck. There are far better ways to protect a stroke survivor in early recovery.

When patients are discharged, family members are often provided with pamphlets explaining how to modify the home environment and information about rehab options, home therapy, community-based programs, and other resources that are specific to their hometown, but they might not receive guides that help them adjust to the changes in emotions, cognition, and behavior that family members may find bewildering. They also may not be informed about the new techniques and electronic devices that are helping survivors regain their motor skills while improving brain "plasticity," its amazing ability to rewire itself after a stroke. I want to provide this information here because it is not readily available elsewhere.

How to Respond to the Changes

Survivors may be impaired in different ways, depending on the severity and location of the damage. Following are common problems that caregivers face.

- *Perception of body impairment.* Survivors tend to ignore the side of their bodies that has become paralyzed or weak. You can help by massaging the affected limb, or having them rub it themselves. Ask them to turn their heads in the direction of the affected side and look in that direction, which they also tend to ignore. If this is so, keep the things they need, such as eyeglasses or food, on the unaffected side of their body to avoid confusion. They also may lack depth and distance perception. You can help by moving furniture and other objects they may bump into or stumble over as they make their way around the house.

- *Lack of awareness of their physical limitations.* Survivors may be unaware that they can no longer perform habitual tasks. They will need to be supervised until they understand what they safely can and cannot do.

- *Confusion.* Stroke patients can lose their bearings easily. You can help by creating a calm environment. Monitor television watching to avoid violence or other disturbing images. Too much auditory stimulation also can be agitating. The combination of people talking, music playing, television blaring, and a phone ringing can make them disoriented. Establishing a routine and sticking to it also helps reduce their confusion.

- *Impaired cognition and language skills.* When communicating, speak slowly, using visual cues, and be patient when waiting for a response. Don't try to guess what the response might be. The survivor needs practice in retrieving words, but it may take time. Ask questions that can be answered with a yes or a no.

- *Fatigue.* Everything is an effort for the survivor, and although movement of the body and stimulation of the mind are important, the real healing takes place during sleep. Irritation is often a sign that that load limit has been reached.

- *Guilt.* A survivor may be overwhelmed with feelings of remorse over the ways a family has been disrupted by the stroke, especially over constantly having to ask others for help. You can ease feelings of helplessness by letting them make whatever decisions won't endanger them, such as when or what they want to eat. A missed meal is not worth fussing over.

- *Depression.* It is only natural that the survivor feels incredibly sad and discouraged over what has happened. When depression slides into immobility, feelings of worthlessness, loss of appetite, or the expression of suicidal thoughts, it is appropriate to seek help from a mental health professional. If an antidepressant is recommended, make sure you consult with a neurologist about the type of medication, because certain kinds of antidepressants are counterproductive for people recovering from stroke.

Rehab and Robotic Breakthroughs

Because of the discovery of the recoverable brain, a revolution is under way in the field of stroke rehabilitation. Some of this transformation is the result of technological developments, but most of it is the result of new procedures that have been studied and found to enhance recovery of motor skills and brain function. I'll describe these procedures in the following list.

- *Constraint-induced movement therapy.* This new technique treats patients whose impaired arm no longer functions by wearing a restraint on the unaffected arm. After an intensive, two-week course of repetitive exercise, patients have regained function, even in arms that were too weak to perform any tasks at the onset of treatment. Neuroimaging also revealed increased activity in the part of the brain that controlled the impaired arm.

- *Transcranial magnetic stimulation.* This noninvasive, painless new therapy uses a device placed on the scalp that passes a brief magnetic pulse, stimulating the cortex or outer part of the brain. In a recent study, after three sessions, patients' motor function improved by as much as 50 percent.

- *Gait training.* Encouraging results have been found in this new procedure, which guides the legs and feet into the proper walking motion on a treadmill, assisted by harness support.

- *The SuperSlow workout.* I found this method of weight training very effective in increasing muscle strength. When reps are done quickly, momentum does part of the work. In slow-motion workouts, the muscles do it all, with the help of a special breathing technique that extends your efforts to the maximum, where real muscle strength is developed. This form of training is also safer for stroke survivors than more vigorous methods of exercise, although every bit as exhausting!

- *RUPERT and other robotic friends are on the way.* RUPERT is short for robotic upper extremity repetitive therapy, a high-tech machine with pneumatic muscles at the shoulder, elbow, and wrist. In studies it has been found to be effective in restoring movement to the arm impaired by a stroke. Like other recent rehab treatments, RUPERT works on the brain, increasing its plasticity. Similar robotic devices are also in development. Right now they are very expensive, but when they can be manufactured at an affordable price, they will save survivors money in the cost of rehab.

6

Walking

———◦———

I HAD NEVER BEEN AFRAID of flying before. In fact, I had enjoyed it, especially the exhilarating feeling I would get on takeoff, when the plane accelerates to a speed that magically lifts it into the air—passengers, baggage, and all. Like so many feelings poststroke, that, too, had changed.

At the Miami airport, as Pat pushed me in my wheelchair toward a tiny, thirty-seat airplane parked at our gate, I started to shake. I had never been afraid of "puddle-jumpers," as I called them, but now my throat started to close up with fear—fear of flying and fear of what lay ahead at my destination. All my emotions had been intensified by the stroke, and this one—anxiety—was especially distressing for me, having always taken pride in my fearlessness.

As I was buckled into my seat, I decided to try something that had helped me in other stressful situations. I closed my eyes and visualized a red carpet being rolled ahead of us down the runway, with angels standing on each side. When we reached liftoff, that image of a red carpet surrounded by angels kept me focused and peaceful all the way to our destination.

When we landed at the little town of Puerto Plata on the northern coast of the island of Hispaniola, all the Dominican nationals aboard the plane started clapping, their traditional way of thanking the pilot. I thought it was a very gracious gesture. Even before I got off the plane, I knew I was going to like these people.

As Pat wheeled me through the open-air island terminal, I immediately felt overdressed in my heavy attire. My workout pants were definitely the wrong pick.

Though the Dominican Republic is not that far south of Florida, the heat was much more intense, and the humidity was so thick I could actually feel the moisture in the air. Pat waved for a porter to pick up our luggage, and we proceeded to the outside curb. I stared in amazement at the unique collection of taxicabs lined up on the dusty street, where drivers were waiting for customers. There were old army jeeps with no tops, battered vans called combis, and VW Beetles with fringe hanging from the rearview mirrors. The drivers were dressed for the heat in sandals and light linen apparel.

Immediately a throng of wannabe drivers surrounded us, each one clamoring to be chosen. My mind was a confused jumble as I tried to sort out these new images and all the voices speaking at once. I was anxious and fearful all over again.

What on earth was I doing here?

In front of one of the vans we spied a man holding up a sign bearing my name. What a welcome sight! Pat waved to him, and he made his way through the sea of drivers. As we were unable to discern his heavily accented English, he communicated his intent to us by pointing to the sign he was holding, and then to us.

"Yes!" we replied, nodding our heads with enthusiasm.

"Buenos días," he said. "I'm Sammy. I drive you to clinic."

He loaded our luggage into his van, then wheeled my chair onto a lift and got me situated in the back of his van. It was a customized vehicle from the late seventies, with a bench sofa in the back and a large window on either side. All that was missing was a shag carpet and Sonny and Cher.

Sammy started the van and turned on the radio. Lively Spanish music set the mood for the ride, and off we went. It seemed as if there was no legal speed limit in the D.R., nor were there dividing lines on our coarse two-lane asphalt road. Hanging on for dear life to the arms of my wheelchair, I settled in for the thirty-minute drive to the Hospital of the Americas Plaza. Nevertheless, I was getting used to being a captive of my circumstances and learning how to go with the flow, even when that flow was so fast that everything out the window became a blur.

The foliage was thick and lush, not like that of some Caribbean islands I had been on. I saw miles of fields of sugarcane, which is a major crop on the island and the raw material for one of its major exports: rum. While I was in the airport terminal, I had noticed that rum also was the island's official beverage, offered in paper shot glasses to the arriving passengers. As we careened along the winding road, I was perplexed and alarmed to observe children and adults walking along the roadside carrying large machetes over their shoulders. Sammy explained to us in gestures and broken English that we shouldn't worry; they were merely workers returning home from the sugarcane fields.

He finally slowed down as we approached the small village where the medical facility was located and drove up to a tall set of iron gates, guarded by soldiers dressed in full fatigues and holding machine guns. Once again I was troubled. After the soldiers had waved us through the gates, Pat asked Sammy, "Why are there gates and soldiers?"

Sammy pointed west. "Over there is Haiti. Not safe. No worries. Safe where you going." Visitors to the Dominican Republic were heavily guarded.

Once we were through the gates, our surroundings changed dramatically. Instead of thatched houses lining the road there were beautifully landscaped grounds with towering palms and bright flowers. Resort accommodations surrounded a plush golf course in the center of the village. It was a stark change from what we had witnessed just before, like walking out of a ghetto into a Disney theme park.

The Hospital of the Americas Plaza was decorated Polynesian style, with shops and restaurants on the first floor and the clinic on the second floor. Pat wheeled me into the elevator, which opened to double glass doors leading to the clinic, where a receptionist was awaiting our arrival. Cadie was a pretty, young Dominican with long, dark hair and a beautiful smile. She spoke English fluently and would be our translator.

Although my treatments would not begin until the following day, Cadie gave us a tour of the facility, orienting me to the various rooms I would encounter during my stay. Each one was dedicated to a specific treatment, depending on a patient's protocol. Nearly all the rooms had large floor-to-ceiling windows with spectacular views of the mountains and the ocean. The clinic was specifically designed so that the patients could focus on a peaceful and positive outlook. It was not long into my stay before I understood the important role that environment plays in recovery.

After our orientation, Sammy drove us to the resort hotel down the street. It was a group of villas, one of them dedicated specifically for patients of the clinic. A bellboy drove us in a golf cart down a brick path to our room. It was neat, clean, and very basic, consisting of tiled floors, two double beds, a dresser, and a television. As we were advised not to drink the tap water, Pat went out to buy some bottled water. Upon her return, she helped me out of my wheelchair and into bed so I could relax from the trip. I longed for a hot shower but knew that this was not possible, since I was unable to stand on my own. As my head hit the pillow, I was so exhausted that I immediately fell asleep.

At about three in the morning, I woke up vomiting and choking. I was lying flat on my back, immobilized, unable even to turn my head. Within seconds I began gagging and gasping for air. Pat jumped out of bed, turned my head, and cleared my air passageway. My neck was weak and limp. Even my eyelids were too weak to open. I was having a seizure. She held me through my convulsions and rubbed my back, telling me in a soothing voice that I would be okay.

Once again, I knew I was at death's door; so did Pat. This time, however, there was no one to call. We had not yet met the doctors or nurses who would be providing my care, and the clinic and the front desk were closed. All we could do was wait. It wasn't long before my convulsions ceased and Pat was able to change my shirt and wash my face. Spent, I passed out and slept till later that morning.

As I look back on that terrifying experience, I realize that my fears about being a patient in a foreign country were not unfounded or exaggerated. I can now appreciate just how vulnerable I had really been following my discharge from the hospital. Had those convulsions happened while I was alone at home, completely immobilized, most likely I would have died. Those angels had been working overtime on my behalf!

I woke up as a bright beam of sunlight burst through the tiny opening between the draperies. "Thank you, God," I whispered. The beam of light was like a message, letting me know I had survived the night and that a new and hopeful day had begun. Pat and I were both eager to begin my treatments. Sammy arrived and loaded me into the van with the automatic wheelchair lift. I hung my head in humiliation as the tourists stared at me inquisitively.

Arriving at the medical plaza, we proceeded into the elevator and to the second floor. Cadie greeted us and took me to a room where I changed into a green surgical top and matching drawstring bottom. She removed my diamond stud earrings and gave them to Pat for safekeeping. After being wheeled into the next room, I was assisted out of my wheelchair and into a comfortable recliner and served my first meal.

Breakfast consisted of two hard-boiled eggs, unbuttered wheat toast, and papaya juice. The server was very polite, though like most of the staff, he did not speak a word of English. Thankfully, his expressions were lovingly clear as he smiled and gestured that I should "eat up."

After breakfast, my vitals were taken and I was started on my first therapy, an intravenous detoxification of heavy metals prepared specifically for my body chemistry. Island music played softly in the background as I sat in a recliner for an hour watching the clear IV bag slowly empty its contents into a vein.

I spent the entire day rolling from room to room, receiving a number of treatments. The most memorable therapy was in an all-white room with a large submarine-looking chamber. In the middle of the room sat a large tank with dials and switches running along the side. It looked like a large steel coffin. A technician in a white jacket was seated on a stool, facing the dials and meters. The back of the tank was open, and a long, flat metal tray extended out from it. As I stared at it in bewilderment, stunned and confused, the staff physician entered the room.

"Good morning, Valerie. My name is Dr. Alcedevez. Just call me 'Dr. A' for short; it will be easier for you to say." He then explained the procedure I was about to undergo.

"Valerie, this is a hyperbaric oxygen chamber. It delivers pressurized oxygen to areas of poor circulation and tissue damage, and it is vital to your recovery. There is nothing to fear. You will not feel or smell anything. You just lie comfortably and breathe normally. We even have a video for you to watch if you'd like. There is a window for you to look out, and someone will always be sitting right here. You'll be in it for one hour two times a day, so just rest and the time will fly by."

I was given a natural liquid valerian to relax me. I lay on the metal tray as they slid me into the tank and then closed the opening behind me. I could hear a drill securing the bolts on the closed steel door. Normally, this would have freaked me

out, but thanks to the valerian I was in la-la land and too tran-
quil to care. Waving to a group of doctors, I relaxed and began
to watch *Terminator 2*. Little did I know that it was one of only
two videos offered, and it was in Spanish to boot!

When my two hours of confinement in the chamber were
over, I heard the drill as it loosened the bolts on the door and
decided that the procedure wasn't too bad. Besides, it gave me
the opportunity to learn some Spanish as well.

"*Hasta la vista*, baby!" I said to Dr. A as I emerged.
Everyone laughed. Oddly, I found that speaking Spanish was
easier for me, poststroke, than speaking English.

In a very short while I grew close to the staff, especially Dr.
A, who monitored all my treatments. He was compassionate
and understood my need for reassurance.

Only a few days had passed since our arrival when an emergency alert was sounded, announcing that Hortense, a category
four hurricane, was rapidly approaching the island. Its 140-
mile-per-hour winds and ravaging rains had lashed Puerto
Rico, some 250 miles southeast of Puerto Plata, causing widespread destruction. Now the storm had taken dead aim at the
small island of Hispaniola, of which the Dominican Republic
occupies the eastern portion. Tourists scrambled to catch
departing flights and evacuate the island before nightfall.

Having worked so hard to get there, and still in the early
stages of my treatment, I did not want to leave. Fortunately, Pat
agreed with my decision to stay and was willing to stick it out
with me. After all, we were from Florida and were used to tropical storms, or so we thought.

In truth, I probably would have stayed even if Pat hadn't.
Imagine boarding a tiny puddle-jumper and getting tossed
around in the sky. I would have been nauseated for days even if
we could evacuate. So we hunkered down.

We knew that a category four hurricane would do damage
and we could lose power, so Pat bought candles, bottled water,

bananas, and peanut butter. That evening the storm came ashore. Furious 130 mile-per-hour winds tore through the island, shredding the bamboo and palms surrounding our villa. We did not have a radio, and the television was useless. Pat kept our draperies closed in case the winds broke the glass. The lights flickered as the power lines were damaged by the heavy winds.

Nevertheless, we felt safe, still protected by those angels. We knew we had not come this far only to be run off by a hurricane. Throughout the night we listened to the crashing of trees and the howling wind as it tore through the hall outside our door. The eye of the hurricane was within twenty-five miles of us when, miraculously, it turned to the northeast, just missing us.

The next morning we saw debris lying everywhere. Cars were stranded in high pools of water, and many trees were down. Everyone was assessing the brutal beating that the high winds and twenty inches of rainfall had inflicted. There were reports of mudslides in the upper regions of the island and in nearby villages. Many people had been victimized. I watched the locals working to clean up the debris and wondered if my driver would be able to get through to pick us up. But Sammy arrived at eight o'clock sharp, waving and asking us if we were okay.

The terrifying experiences we had survived since our arrival—first the seizure and then the hurricane—only fortified my resolve, strangely enough. Nothing could stop me from going on with my recovery! I resumed my treatments, and as the days went by, I continued to show signs of improvement. I could have received most of these treatments in the United States, but at that time live stem cell injections were available only at an offshore clinic. They were the primary reason why I had gone to the trouble and expense of going to the Dominican Republic. Stem cell injections had been used around the globe with great success for more than sixty years. In spite of the promising results and a long and impressive track record, however, at that time the United States was not offering stem cell therapy as an approved or even a legal method of treatment.

Even today few people realize, as I didn't then, that stem cells are available and effective from sources other than a human. Mine were from a lamb. In their embryonic stage, cells of animal species are identical to human cells until the time of species differentiation. In other words, a lamb embryo will look like a human embryo until it becomes old enough to differentiate into a lamb. These young embryonic cells can be harvested and given by injection to humans.

Before my first injection, I was comforted to find out that a team of doctors from around the world came to the clinic regularly to share their knowledge and expertise with the local staff. Even so, before I received my injections, I looked up at Dr. A. with grave concern.

"Are you sure?" I asked. I was afraid and needed reassurance.

He lowered the syringe to his side and looked at me with compassion and understanding. "Yes, I'm sure," he said with confidence. This became our little ritual. Before each injection I would ask, "Are you sure?" and he would always give me the same answer.

The day after my first injection, Dr. A. asked me how I felt. Knowing that the stem cells came from a lamb, I looked up innocently at him and the nurses and answered, "Baaaahhhh."

Everyone was silent until I gave them a mischievous smile, and they realized I was playing with them. We all broke into laughter.

Every day I continued to improve. The treatments were working! I could move my left hand and left arm more freely, and my left leg was getting stronger. In addition to the physical improvements, my mental function had dramatically improved. My mind felt clearer, almost as though a fog was being lifted.

At the end of the first week, Pat and I were invited to have dinner with Cadie, our interpreter, and her fiancé at her home. She lived in an apartment building outside the tourist area, so we arranged for a cab to take us. Leaving the heavily guarded village was, once again, like entering a different world. We shared the roads with donkeys and small cars that were so beaten up they looked like they had been in a demolition derby. I even saw one car without any doors. The harsh realities of poverty were evident everywhere. People watched us through the iron gates of their homes as we passed by. It was all I could do not to stare back.

Cadie invited us into her apartment and asked us to pardon the confusion, as more than one family shared the small space. The living conditions were unlike anything I had ever seen. A gas line dangled loose over the kitchen sink, where drinking water boiled in a large tin pot. A clothesline was strung out the kitchen window, with clothes flapping in the warm island breeze.

After a dinner of rice and beans, Cadie served us canned flan, a delicacy she had been saving for a special occasion. As we sat around the living room, she and her fiancé talked about their lives and ambitions. They spoke of the United States as if it were paradise. It was heartbreaking for me to realize that they dreamed of what I took for granted: owning a car, living in their own space, or just having air-conditioning. It really opened my eyes to how fortunate I was in spite of my medical condition.

As the evening drew to a close, darkness filled the room while the electricity began to flicker off and on. Cadie calmly lit several candles, as if this happened every night—which it did. She explained that the government deliberately turned the power off and on like this throughout the city to punish the people who hooked up electricity without paying. Barbaric as this was, she and the others had grown accustomed to the inconvenience and had learned to adjust to it.

When it was time for us to go, Cadie called another cab for

us. Only the moon and an occasional passing car lit the dark streets as Pat and I sat silently in the backseat of the taxi, pondering the experience we had just shared.

The next day, word of our visit spread through the clinic, and Sammy wasted no time in inviting us to meet his family. We graciously accepted, but explained that we could not stay long. The next day, after treatment, he drove us to his home, about thirty minutes from the clinic. As we drew near, the streets narrowed and we approached a cluster of small, ramshackle, wooden homes. He lived on one of these narrow streets, where children were playing, awaiting our arrival. Sammy parked the van on the street just outside the front door. He held my arm as I walked with my cane up the steps to his house. The front door was so short we had to lower our heads as we entered. Inside, the entire family had gathered—his wife and children plus his brothers, sisters, and parents. We were greeted by their warm, smiling faces welcoming us. Sammy introduced us to each member of his entire extended family. He was the only one who spoke English, however, so our visit was brief, though full of smiles.

What a powerful healing experience this was for me. I'd left the States feeling like a disabled, second-class citizen. But Sammy's family was so honored to have me in their home that I felt like royalty. This gracious family had lifted my spirits and helped to restore my injured self-worth.

As that first week came to an end, Pat had to return home. Like me, she had grown to admire and appreciate this beautiful country and its people. We had shared some memorable times, and her dry sense of humor had kept me smiling, able to see the lighter side of things. I was going to miss having her around. Before leaving, she made arrangements for one of the nurses from the clinic to stay with me.

Mail started to arrive from home. I was so anxious to receive word from my family and friends, and the cost of making or receiving international phone calls was outrageous. Not that it really mattered; the only viable form of communication for me was letter writing. E-mail would have been wonderful, but in 1996 it was not as readily available as it is now.

The staff noted my strong desire to receive mail, so my nurse took me to an office in the medical plaza and pointed out a fax machine I could use for a small fee. As I realized what was being offered me, I was like a kid on Christmas Day. I was so excited! Each morning during my hour-long chelation session, I would prepare faxes to send out. It wasn't long before I was receiving one or more a day—inspiring and encouraging messages, get-well wishes, silly jokes, cartoons, and word of how my Alex was doing.

The medical staff and doctors were extremely sensitive and comforting, but my loneliness weighed heavily on me and I longed to be home. Yet, each day as I continued the treatments, I was encouraged to see changes as my body healed.

Supported by therapists on each side of me, I practiced standing and walking on my own. At times they even danced with me to liven things up. The nurses were salsa-dancing experts. Whether or not they had music to accompany them, it was in their bones. I had always been a very good dancer, but now I was out of my league. It was all I could do just to keep from stepping on their toes.

By the second week, I was able to stand on my own and walk a few steps without falling. I was making monumental improvement, although I still used my cane, but now I felt steady and was much better balanced. As the days passed, I could feel my left side continue to gain strength. A medical miracle was happening right before my eyes. How I wished my therapists back at the hospital in Florida could see my progress. They would be so thrilled!

Dr. Christa, the chief medical director of the clinic, heard of my remarkable progress and invited me to visit her at her home, about two hours from the clinic, in Santo Domingo. She provided a round-trip bus ticket for me, assuring me it would be safe to travel that way, and promised to pick me up upon my arrival.

It was a clear, sunny day as I boarded the open-air bus for the trip south to the capital, one that revealed sights both breathtaking and heartbreaking. In contrast with the beautiful countryside framed by mountains and blue water, there were thatched homes and dirt yards where children played. The Dominican Republic didn't seem to have a middle class. People were either very wealthy or incredibly poor, but one thing was consistent: they were all loving and gracious.

When I arrived in Santo Domingo, Dr. Christa was there to greet me just as she had promised. She drove me through the city to the first upper-class residential area I had seen. We drove through a gated entrance and to her home. From the third-floor balcony, I could see fields of banana trees with a few marijuana plants growing between them. Amid the plants I spotted a white rabbit eating the plants. I smiled, wondering how it might feel after eating marijuana leaves all day.

While dinner was being prepared, Dr. Christa gave me a tour of her beautiful home and the guest quarters where her partner, Mr. Freedman, lived. He was the engineer who had designed and built the hyperbaric oxygen chamber for the clinic. I had seen him through the window of the chamber every day, but this was the first time we had been introduced.

Dr. Christa commented on how well my treatment was going and then said, "I read in your chart that you were a golfer before your stroke. Would you like to join us tomorrow morning for a round at our club?"

"*Sí, muchas gracias,*" I answered. My eyes welled up with tears, thinking how just months before I had been in the ICU, dangling between life and death. Now I was being invited to go to a golf course. This was, for me, a real indication that I was finally beginning to regain my life.

The next day we all went to the clubhouse for an early

breakfast. Afterward, Dr. Christa drove me around in her golf cart and gave me a tour of the course. It was unlike anything I had ever seen. Surrounded by mountains and a jungle of thick, tropical foliage, it appeared to be a golf course in the middle of a jungle. The clubhouse had no exterior walls and was set on a cliff overlooking the eighteenth hole. It looked like a Tarzan movie set. I watched from the golf cart as Dr. Christa and Mr. Freedman teed off, and it was all I could do not to grab a nine-iron and punch the next ball. Watching them, I knew it wouldn't be long before I'd be back, swinging my golf clubs with determination.

The lovely weekend passed quickly, and I returned to the clinic to continue my treatments. Day after day, I remained under constant care as I underwent my routine of scheduled treatments.

During my last week, my father flew down for a quick visit. I was looking forward to seeing him again. My dad was an inter-esting man. He had a heart of gold when it came to his fellow man, as long as his fellow man didn't cross him or get in his way. He was handsome and well dressed, and his good-hearted-ness made him irresistible to the ladies and easy to forgive; but he packed a punch of prejudice against everything that wasn't Caucasian or American. I'm not certain why Dad was that way. Perhaps his own father's John Wayne-ish, tough-guy facade had something to do with it. "Pappy," as we called our grandfather, would often share stories of driving a tank in World War II and would proudly show off his war scars. If Pappy had a softer side, I never saw it in the thirteen years I knew him before he died.

A natural-born salesman, my dad could sell anything from property to dreams. His customers warmed to his humor and practical jokes, and many of them became friends. Dad was involved in so many businesses in his lifetime, I eventually lost track. He was a true entrepreneur who never gave up.

He made the mark as a father in most ways but was absent in others. For him, like many men of his generation, providing materially for the family was a greater priority than providing for our emotional needs. He would join us for church at Easter and at Christmas, but nothing was a sure thing.

During my childhood, he was my hero and I was a daddy's girl. He would never admit it, but I often felt that he favored me over my sisters. He and I went fishing and camping together. He even taught me to shoot a rifle, skeet-shoot with a shotgun, and load buckshot in a .357 Magnum. I became a skilled marksman in no time, even winning shooting competitions over the male contestants. And he taught me to drive a stick shift in his Jeep before I was ten years old, showing me how to work the clutch to climb steep hills.

As I grew up, I admired cars more and more, especially the finer fast ones, such as Ferraris and Maseratis. Some say I was the son he never had, but I was simply a tomboy who loved adventure and thrills. Throughout my childhood, my dad could do no wrong in my eyes, but in my teens, when I discovered his unfaithfulness to my mother, he fell from the pedestal I had put him on. Though he was no longer my idol, I learned to accept him for who he was. I never questioned his love for me, and no matter what, I continued to love him very much.

Just knowing that Dad was coming to see me was very exciting. Sammy drove me to the airport to pick him up. It was Friday afternoon, and my treatments for the week were over, so we went to the beach. It was the first time I'd been there, and it was more beautiful than I had imagined. Palms trees and cabanas lined the beaches. We sat under a tiki hut and had a cool island beverage while enjoying the sights. Swimsuit tops were optional, and Dad seemed very content watching the sunbathers who opted not to wear one. It was a beautiful day, and I enjoyed relaxing and being with my father. He took me to dinner that evening, where our conversation remained light; we talked of the weather, his business, and his latest girlfriend. I remember wanting to know but failing to ask him why he never came to be with me in the hospital.

When it was time for him to leave on Sunday morning, I rode with Sammy when he drove Dad to the airport to catch his departing flight. I kissed him good-bye and gave him a big hug. As he walked to the small plane waiting on the island runway, he turned and waved.

"I love you, B!" he shouted. "B" was the nickname he had given me as a little girl and that he had called me ever since. Then he turned and boarded the plane. On the drive back to the clinic, I wondered why we hadn't discussed his absence, as it was so heavy on my heart. Maybe it was a wound neither of us wanted to open. All I know is that I never asked him, and he never offered information that satisfied me.

While it does not serve to excuse him, over the years I came to learn that when Dad was faced with the thought of my dying, he froze in denial rather than run to my side. Regardless, I still felt abandoned. Neither my mother nor my father was truly present for me during this most critical time of my life. My mother and I were distant emotionally, and my father, by miles. For many years this was, and still can be, difficult to think about.

A very good therapist advised me to write about my feelings, expressing how deeply this had hurt me.

"Even if you never share these letters with your parents, writing down your feelings will help you release the disappointment and hurt," she advised me. After years of therapy and spiritual growth I was able to forgive them.

My last weekend at the clinic finally arrived, and my sister Angie and a mutual friend, Bonnie, flew down to escort me home. Once again, it was my big sister to the rescue. I couldn't wait to see her face when I showed her the progress I had made. Bartering with one of the locals, I arranged for a horse-drawn carriage to pick them up at the hotel in the morning and bring them to the clinic.

That evening my doctor made reservations at a special

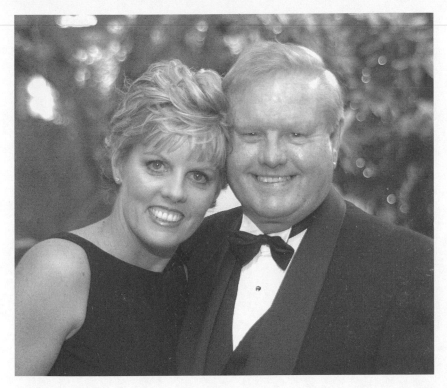

Dad and me

restaurant that was famous for its unique location—in a huge
tree. The restaurant sat high above the ground, with lions and
other exotic animals on display in cages below. A large table
was waiting for us, and after everyone was seated, they toasted
my recovery and congratulated me on all my hard work. While
I had much more physical therapy ahead of me, the treatments
had been very successful. Angie and Bonnie enjoyed the rest of
the evening with me as we played and laughed endlessly, pre-
tending to smoke the expensive cigars that were given to
everyone after dinner. We even ventured down to the lions'
den below for a closer look.

The remainder of the weekend we prepared for my return
home. Angie and Bonnie shopped for souvenirs, while I gathered mementos and gifts for the clinic staff.

Once again I had bonded with a group of special people, and I knew that I would miss them. Each person had been instrumental in my survival and recovery. They continue to hold a special place in my heart and memories today.

I was going home again—not like that first time out of the hospital following my stroke. This homecoming was going to be different. I was going to reclaim the ground I had lost to this stroke. It has been said that it is not what others call us that defines us as people, but it is what we answer to. I was no longer willing to be defined by labels of "infirm," "handicapped," or "limited."

I was now ready to rebuild my life, not just my body.

Hyperbaric Oxygen Therapy: "The Best-Kept Medical Secret"

*We run on a double standard in this country. Show me
a double-blind, placebo-controlled study for hip
replacements and then I'll talk to you about the need
for these studies in the use of HBOT for the brain.*

—William S. Maxfield, M.D., F.A.C.N.M.;
board-certified in radiology, nuclear medicine,
and hyperbaric medicine; cofounder of the
American Board of Hyperbaric Medicine

W HEN STROKE SURVIVORS see the amazing recovery I made
from a stroke that should have killed or permanently disabled me, they always ask the same question: "How did you do
it?" I tell them that although I credit many different kinds of
therapy, the most important is hyperbaric oxygen therapy
(HBOT). It is also a predominantly safe and minimally invasive
procedure, is approved by the FDA, and has been successfully
used in clinical treatment in the United States and other countries for more than fifty years.

The way hyperbaric (pronounced hyper-*bair*-ic) treatment
works is very simple: it gives the brain a large dose of oxygen, the
lack of which caused the stroke in the first place. During a brain
attack, the damage is described as being like an atomic bomb. In
the epicenter the neurons are dead, but fanning out from it is an
area called the penumbra, where the neurons are damaged but
still alive. These idling neurons can be revived by oxygen, delivered under pressure, which pushes the oxygen into the body fluids.

Normally, the air we breathe is about 20 percent oxygen, depending on where we live. In HBOT, 100 percent pure oxygen is administered through a chamber in which the air is pressurized, much like in an airplane cabin, which increases the amount of oxygen the body takes in to many times its normal amount. In the brain, this jolt of oxygen reactivates idling nerve cells, stimulating the body to produce new blood vessels that begin to deliver more blood to the damaged tissue. HBOT also reduces inflammation caused by the dead cells and increases what is called plasticity—the amazing ability of other parts of the brain to take over the functions of the area where cells have died.

The quicker these damaged cells receive HBOT, the better the results. In one study of 152 patients treated with HBOT within the first fours following the onset of a stroke, 38 were discharged the next day for outpatient treatment. Another study demonstrated that this treatment could significantly decrease mortality if given within the first three days after a stroke.

The opportunity for using HBOT is hardly ever available during the acute phase of a stroke, which is unfortunate, because the

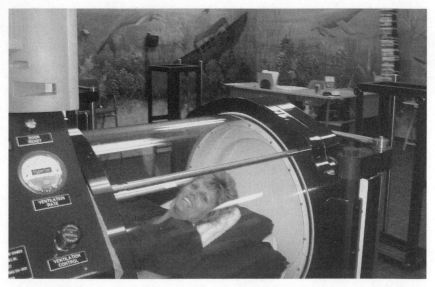

Me in a hyperbaric chamber

longer the damaged cells have been dormant, the more reluctant they are to wake up. As a result, most hyperbaric treatments are given five days a week for a month or longer before improvement begins. But when HBOT works, neurons that have been dormant for months or even years can regain their activity and begin functioning.

Why isn't HBOT standard procedure for treating stroke? I asked that question to top experts in the field of neurology and hyperbaric medicine, and this is what they told me:

- The vast majority of medical doctors have been taught that brain damage is irreversible.

- HBOT is seldom taught in medical schools.

- HBOT has been tested by only a few randomized, double-blind, placebo-controlled clinical trials, the current so-called gold standard of proof.

- HBOT is used in hospitals to treat a number of other medical conditions, but not stroke.

- With rare exceptions, HBOT is not covered by insurance. Some doctors are under contractual obligations with insurance companies that won't even allow them to recommend HBOT to their patients.

- For decades, HBOT has been discredited by celebrities making outrageous claims about its benefits, such as calling it the fountain of youth.

- Because HBOT can't be patented, there's no money to be made in marketing it.

Resistance to the Concept of the Recoverable Brain

Up to ten years ago, the established medical opinion was that nothing could be done about brain tissue that had been damaged by a stroke. Since then, researchers have taken advantage of new technologies and as a result a number of studies have been published that prove that some brain cells can regenerate. Even though many of these studies have been conducted by mainstream medical researchers and published in respected mainstream medical journals, many physicians still cling to the information they were taught in medical school. They continue to insist that brain cells do not regenerate and even discredit the doctors who say they do.

This resistance to change within the medical community remains a major hurdle to overcome before the use of hyperbaric oxygen therapy becomes clinically available to the millions of people in this country who might possibly benefit from it.

A Lack of Knowledge about HBOT

Wrong information about HBOT is not the only obstacle to its becoming a mainstream treatment for a stroke. No information at all is another: only twelve medical schools in this country teach hyperbaric medicine as part of the curriculum. As a result, the vast majority of medical doctors don't accept HBOT simply because they haven't heard about it. And those who have may even call it quackery. For doctors who have witnessed the benefits of HBOT in the patients they treat, this response is frustrating and hard to understand.

Richard A. Neubauer, M.D., was one of those independent thinkers who are way ahead of their times. He was in the forefront of hyperbaric medicine since 1972, and took much of the flak from unbelievers. I was fortunate to be able to interview him for this book just weeks before his untimely death in June 2007.

"Oxygen is too simple, and that's the problem," he told me. "It's all around us, so it's overlooked. I recently saw a one-hour program on stroke on TV, and the word 'oxygen' never came up!

People tell me, 'Oxygen is cheap, it's everywhere, and you get it for nothing just by breathing it in. How do you know that giving it under pressure does any good?' "

The nuclear physicist Edward Teller, Ph.D., the father of the hydrogen bomb, had a stroke in 1995, and he recovered his short-term memory after being treated with HBOT at Dr. Neubauer's clinic in Lauderdale-by-the-Sea, Florida. Teller explained to Dr. Neubauer how the treatment works from Teller's point of view as a physicist: Because oxygen is a gas, it is subject to all the gas laws of physics. According to Henry's Law, if you increase the pressure of a gas, it will be directly increased in whatever takes it in—in HBOT, the cerebrospinal fluid—delivering free molecular oxygen at the tissue level for immediate metabolic use. Then Teller added, "This is far too simple for the average doctor to understand."

The resistance that is common in the United States does not exist in other parts of the world, where HBOT is used to treat more than seventy-three medical conditions, including stroke. It is widely practiced in the United Kingdom, Europe, Russia, South America, and Asia. In China alone, a hundred thousand people are treated each year in hyperbaric oxygen chambers that accommodate up to thirty-six patients who receive oxygen by mask or hood. It is used in conjunction with acupuncture and traditional herbal medicine as a very cost-effective approach to treatment.

To date, physicians from around the world have published about thirty thousand papers in the medical literature on the use of hyperbaric medicine, and the studies keep pouring in. With the rapid rise of an aging population, whose members are more susceptible to a stroke, the time is long overdue for physicians in the United States to learn about the appropriate use of HBOT. Likewise, as the war in Iraq continues, U.S. doctors should consider the benefits of HBOT in treating injured soldiers for traumatic brain injury and in helping to prevent the need for amputation.

Visualizing the Functioning Brain

For twenty years, Dr. Neubauer used an advanced version of an imaging procedure called single photon emission computerized tomography (SPECT) to find dormant cells in a patient's brain that are capable of being reactivated and to document their response to HBOT. Early forms of SPECT cameras had been around for a long time, but the technique soon dropped out of favor with the inventions of the CT scan and the MRI. But the new, high-resolution SPECT cameras are faster and provide clearer results than previous SPECT scans, and they have a great advantage over CTs and MRIs in that they can show how the brain functions by providing color-coded images that demonstrate where, whether, and how much neural activity is taking place. Red, for instance, indicates oxygen-rich, normal function, while yellow indicates oxygen-starved brain tissue.

Experience convinced Dr. Neubauer that the best way to measure the efficacy of hyperbaric oxygen therapy is to use patients as their own control, using the same measurements in each scan before and after HBOT. Over the years he collected a mountain of data at his Ocean Hyperbaric Center, where every patient is given a SPECT scan before beginning treatment as well as additional scans during the course of treatment to objectively mark a patient's progress. Nine times out of ten, he found that the before-and-after scans correlated with the patient's physical and mental improvement, which has proved to be effective in a large number of patients. Multiplied by similar results in thousands of brain-injured patients treated worldwide, these tests provide a massive amount of positive and compelling data for the use of HBOT. But these informally collected data don't meet the requirements for a randomized, placebo-controlled, double-blind clinical trial and so aren't considered as proof of HBOT's effectiveness as a stroke recovery treatment.

A Lack of "Acceptable" Studies
for HBOT

The fact that a drug or a therapy works in a significant number patients is no longer good enough in the eyes of the FDA, the NIH, and the AMA. Ever since World War II, the only acceptable proof has been the double-blind, randomized, placebo-controlled trial. In the United States, this kind of study is mandatory for the approval of a new drug or a treatment, and it's unlikely that this requirement will change anytime soon.

That said, only 17 percent of the medications, interventions, and surgical procedures approved and reimbursed by Medicare have ever been subjected to this kind of test. Had the trials been necessary in the past, open-heart surgery, angioplasty, organ transplants, and the smallpox vaccine may never have been developed, and aspirin would probably not be available at the corner drugstore. There are simply too many situations in medicine, including any kind of pediatric treatment, where the double-blind method of giving placebos to half of the patients in a study is not only unethical but also unthinkable.

William S. Maxfield, M.D., is a radiologist and pioneer in the field of nuclear medicine, with more than fifty years of clinical practice, including nineteen years of hyperbaric oxygen medicine. He has been reading Dr. Neubauer's SPECT scans for many years and finds them extremely useful in following and monitoring response in HBOT. Dr. Maxfield first became familiar with hyperbaric oxygen medicine while serving in the U.S. Navy as a member of the Plutonium Decontamination Team and a teacher of nuclear medicine in the navy's training program at Bethesda Naval Hospital in Maryland. He has been following the strange history of the use of HBOT in the military ever since.

In the early 1960s the only place where people in the United States could get this treatment was in a military hospital, where aviators and divers received it for altitude and decompression sickness. When it was discovered that hyperbaric treatments were also good for a host of other medical conditions, including wound care, the program was expanded to operating theaters in both Europe and the United States. Civilians as well as people in the military received treatment in these military facilities, the most famous case being Jessica McClure, a little girl who in 1987 fell into a well and, after receiving HBOT, made an amazing recovery from wounds and brain injury caused by oxygen deprivation. This treatment continued to play an important role in military medicine throughout the Vietnam War years and into the 1980s. As late as 1989, use of HBOT was described in the journal *Military Medicine* as being "a powerful modality" and "of extreme interest" to the U.S. military forces.

"I cannot believe our injured soldiers coming home from the war on terrorism are not receiving HBOT," says Dr. Maxfield. "For all those years military medicine was a leader in hyperbaric oxygen treatment. Now, when they need it most, I believe they may have one chamber operating. Why is HBOT bypassed in the military today?"

Dr. Maxfield is not the only medical doctor in the field of HBOT who is mystified. He and a number of his colleagues recently attended a conference sponsored by the U.S. Congress, where they spoke at a meeting called "Traumatic Brain Injury: The Signature Wound of the War on Terrorism."

Dr. Maxfield continued, "We talked about the history of HBOT in the military, how in the past it had always led the way in promoting its use, and why the military and the Veterans Administration should be using it for these brain-injured soldiers. Because of all the headlines today about what the war is doing to these kids, one of the articles we took to the meeting was from China, called 'Evaluation of Hyperbaric for Neuropsychiatric Disorders Following Traumatic Brain Injury.' In the study they used SPECT scans before and after HBOT, just like we have done at Dr. Neubauer's Ocean Hyperbaric Center. To date, however, nothing has come out of the meeting about using HBOT for these diseases. There's a wall of silence about this treatment. It's why I call HBOT the best-kept medical secret in this country."

Breaking Down the Wall

This is the information age, and in spite of all the restrictions imposed on physicians by the randomized, double-blind, placebo-controlled clinical trial, it's impossible for anyone or any group to stop the flood of data and studies about the recoverable brain. The problem with living in this age, however, is the availability of *too much* information, and it's all but impossible even for the most dedicated readers—and even doctors—to be aware of it all. The following is a sampling of recent studies they may have missed.

- The first unequivocal confirmation of the recoverable brain came out of Johns Hopkins Hospital, where a breast cancer patient had a bone marrow transplant from a male donor. When she died, neurons with male chromosomes were found in her brain.

- In England more than a thousand patients with cerebrovascular disease were treated with HBOT, with an improvement ranging from 40 percent to 100 percent.

- In China, 310 patients with neuropsychiatric disorders following traumatic brain injury were treated twice with HBOT and given both CT and SPECT scans before each treatment. More than 70 percent of the patients were clinically improved, and SPECT was found to be much more sensitive than CT as a diagnostic tool.

- Data show that HBOT increases the body's stem cell population by a factor of eight. This increase might help explain the rapid healing that can take place after HBOT.

Additional studies are referred to in the resources section at the back of this book.

Insurance Reimbursement Problems for HBOT

At one time, the FDA and the Centers for Medicare and Medicaid Services (CMS) approved the use of HBOT for a neurological condition (cerebral edema, or swelling), but why it was taken off the list of treatments approved for insurance reimbursement is another mystery. Today the CMS has a list of twenty-two "off-label" indications for use of HBOT that are not approved and therefore not covered by insurance. Precedents for HBOT use in neurologic conditions other than stroke are being set, however. In Texas insurance companies cannot deny coverage for HBOT for brain injuries. A patient sued Blue Cross/Blue Shield of Florida and was awarded full reimbursement for HBOT that cleared her symptoms of multiple sclerosis, plus payment of additional HBOT she might need. This coverage, however, is limited to hyperbaric oxygen therapy administered in a hospital.

In 1989 the federal government made a change in the Medicaid law for treating children, mandating states to provide services "necessary to correct or ameliorate" conditions. Previously, the law covered only treatments deemed "medically necessary." Because of this revised wording, and the lobbying efforts of parents of brain-damaged children across the country, a dozen states have already changed their reimbursement policy to cover HBOT for children, and many lawsuits seeking similar changes have been filed in other states. Some private health plans now also cover HBOT for children. An Internet group called Medicaid for HBOT (www.groups.yahoo.com/group/medicaid forhbot) is promoting the use of this treatment for children in every state in the county.

Unfortunately, if you're an adult, the federal mandate for children does not apply. No hyperbaric chamber is FDA-approved for treating adults with neurological conditions. Exceptions do exist, but giving an "off-label" treatment requires approval by the family and the hospital's research board. These exceptions are made only in cases where a life is at stake and nothing else will work, and the treatment won't be covered by insurance. But even if the patient's life is saved and his condition improves, there's no proof that the oxygen therapy worked.

Nevertheless, the word is spreading into mainstream medical circles about the importance of treating a stroke with HBOT. Several years ago, three major hospitals that provide on-site oxygen therapy did a study, "Hyperbaric oxygen in the treatment of patients with cerebral stroke, brain trauma, and neurologic disease," which concluded that the results were "promising and warrant further investigation." Unfortunately, these hospitals still don't treat stroke patients with HBOT. Hopefully, that day will come soon.

The First Clinical Trial for HBOT

James F. Toole, M.D., is the president of the International Stroke Society and a professor of neurology at the Bowman Medical Center at Wake Forest University in Winston-Salem, North Carolina. He has an opinion about clinical trials that many doctors share. "Physicians try to save lives, and if we're saving lives we're not going to randomize. It's like saying, 'Let's do a prospective randomized trial on parachute jumping. Half of them will have parachutes and the other half won't.' If you know something works, it's unethical not to use it. In the case of HBOT, we are not certain that [it] is effective, and so I believe a trial is necessary to prove whether it is a valuable part of managing persons with an acute stroke."

As a naval aviation medical doctor during the Korean War, Dr. Toole took training in hyper- and hypobaric medicine. "We would send guys up in the sky where the air pressure was low and they'd have to get oxygen, and we would send them to look for mines and missing aircraft under the ocean where the pressure is high. I saw that those pressure differences had huge effects on brain function. Still, you can't just say you *know* it works, you have to prove it, and these days, the only way you can do that is by a randomized trial."

Dr. Toole is proposing a study in which the doctors don't know which patients participating in the study are receiving HBOT and which are not. Half of them would be given pressurized oxygen and the other half would get plain air. He says, "It is my fervent hope that we will find the answer and that it will prove to be effective."

Where Can I Get HBOT?

This is the second most frequently asked question I hear from stroke survivors. If they can't go to their nearest hospital to receive HBOT, where *can* they go? The only answer I can give them at this point is to go abroad, as I did, or to a freestanding center in the United States. There are many of these centers around the country, but people need to be very careful in choosing one. Aside from being checked by a local fire inspector, they are not regulated, and if a strict protocol is not followed, HBOT can be dangerous. A pressure within the chamber that rises above the amount determined by the protocol can cause severe toxicity, and wearing anything metal, or even clothing that is not all-cotton, while receiving treatment can cause a fire.

Even though an HBOT center may claim to be run by a physician, he or she may not be on the premises. Not everyone in a white jacket with a name tag on it is a medical doctor. People can go on the Internet and search for a center near their home, but they need to make sure that stroke is treated there, with a physician on the premises. I have looked at many of these Web sites and notice that the centers where a medical doctor supervises the treatments make a point of saying so. In the resources section in the back of this book is a list of HBOT centers that treat stroke and that are supervised by medical doctors, information I have gathered from the Internet. To my knowledge, such a list does not exist anywhere else but in this book.

"It's All About the Money"

Simply said, the major reason for hyperbaric oxygen therapy being "the best-kept medical secret" is probably the most obvious one: profit. Large amounts of money can't be made by developing a treatment that can't be patented. The following explanation was provided by Dr. Neubauer at the conclusion of our interview:

> If drug companies were ever able to create a pill or a drug with the ability to cross the blood-brain barrier and saturate the cerebrospinal fluid with oxygen, reactivate dormant, idling neurons, and create new capillary growth, thus healing the brain, it would be considered one of the greatest advancements that medicine has ever seen. Such a discovery would be worth billions of dollars a year to the manufacturer. Such a discovery already exists, and its cost-effectiveness is phenomenal. Instead of earning drug companies billions, it would save patients and their families billions, as well as afford a quality of life to people for whom standard medicine has relinquished all hope. Oxygen is God's gift to man, and hyperbaric oxygen is simply a more efficient delivery system for one of the most crucial elements to life on earth.

Whether a brain has been injured in an accident, in combat, from shaken baby syndrome, or from a disease such as stroke, all these tragedies share the same pathology—some cells are dead while others are recoverable—and hyperbaric oxygen therapy has been found to be an effective way of returning these injured cells to effective functioning. One of my major goals in writing this book is to provide information straight from the source— medical doctors at the top of their field—to help promote the use of hyperbaric medicine in this country.

7

Letting Go

───◆───

IRETURNED FROM THE DOMINICAN REPUBLIC exhilarated and with renewed hope. With every step, I felt liberated and joyful, like a toddler taking her first steps. Despite the cane I had to rely on for support, I was standing on my own two feet. Inch by inch, I watched with fascination as my feet slowly moved across the floor. My wheelchair was no longer a fixture in my life and was necessary only when I needed to travel longer distances. When I graduated from a three-pronged cane to a single cane, it was the equivalent of leaving elementary school and moving directly to high school.

My cane was no ordinary, run-of-the-mill kind. It was custom-made of mahogany and had an antique glass doorknob for a handle. I figured that as long as I had to use a cane, it was going to look classy. But as remarkable as it was, from the moment I began using it, I already envisioned framing it one day and hanging it on my wall as a trophy of my resolve. I was putting my faith and courage to the test. No longer would I allow myself to be defined by other people's expectations, or lack thereof.

My progress gave me hope and fueled my determination to reclaim my identity and rebuild my life. Nothing was going to

149

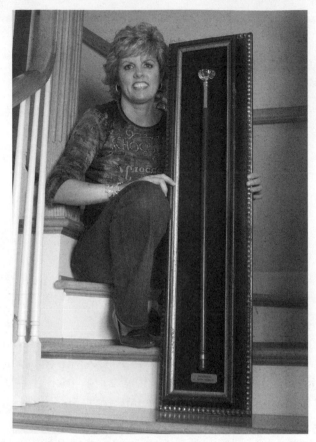

Holding my framed cane

stand in the way of resurrecting the woman I was before the stroke. My hoop dreams were that one day I would walk back into my business office, sit behind my glorious mahogany desk, pick up the telephone, and reconnect with my clients. As a result, I was driven to diligently continue follow-up treatments that I had begun at the clinic: hyperbaric oxygen, nutrition regime, homeopathic treatments, acupuncture—the works.

But restoration of my life, as it had been, was not to be. I began to realize that no matter how much I wanted it otherwise, it was improbable that I would return to a career in finance. My physical challenges were still great. My speech was slurred and difficult to understand, while the most ominous obstacle I faced was that I could no longer add or subtract accurately. The stroke had severely injured my math skills. I felt that I was doing very well to be able to calculate small purchases and transactions. In truth, whenever I shopped for groceries or medications, I became nervous, uncertain that I had enough money to cover my purchase. I would fork over a twenty-dollar bill, or even a fifty, and hope it was adequate to cover my bill. I had to trust that I would be given the correct change.

One time, when I handed the grocery clerk a twenty-dollar bill, she looked at me and said, "It's $21.98; you're short $1.98." I froze, not knowing what to do. The idea of putting something back did not occur to me. After a long pause the clerk could tell something was wrong, as could the other people waiting in line. A very kind person behind me handed the clerk two dollars. I left the store, humiliated.

Resuming my career would have required much more than calculation skills. My brain simply could not handle the complexities it once had performed so adeptly. My diminished speech was another major factor in my recognizing that I would never return to my work. How could I ever conduct business on the telephone? It was challenging enough talking to people face-to-face, much less over the phone.

With great anguish I began to realize that for me there could be no going back; I would have to find another way to move forward.

In the meantime, I had some serious financial decisions to make. My only income was from my disability insurance, which was just enough to cover my house payment and electric bill. I adored my beautiful house, the first I'd ever called my own. I'd had my eye on it for years before it became available. The designer, who had remodeled it, decided to move just as I was in the market to buy. It had been perfect timing. It was a harsh awakening when I realized that I could no longer afford to keep my house. Without any additional income, there was no way I could maintain the standard of living to which I'd grown accustomed. I had to make some drastic changes without delay.

My house was put on the market, and it sold within a week to the first person who looked at it. As soon as the house sold, flyers were mailed, announcing I would have an estate sale.

As it was October, and one of my favorite holidays, Halloween, was just around the corner, I decided to have one last party in my home. Close friends agreed to invite all the guests and arrange for the food. I was in charge of decorating the house. Within a few days it resembled a haunted mansion. On Halloween night the front yard was covered with styrofoam tombstones, surrounded by a sea of misty fog, created by dry ice, floating along the ground. Fake spider webs were strung along the front porch, while a fan blew the curtains out the second-floor windows. A sound track of eerie organ music wafted out of the house, while a strobe light intermittently lit up the darkened rooms. It was spooky—and so was I, wearing a scary mask.

As the party guests arrived, I sat quietly on the front porch swing, holding a bucket of candy and waiting for the last of the trick-or-treaters. Some of my guests were unknown to me and had been invited by my friends. One of them, Missy, took the time to have a conversation with me, really listening so she could understand what I was saying. I learned that she was on partial disability because of fibromyalgia. We hit it off right away and became good friends. Besides having physical challenges in common, Missy was great support. She even helped me with my estate sale the following weekend.

That Saturday, I sold everything in the house that I couldn't fit into my car or in the small U-haul I had rented. Everything was priced to sell quickly. I wanted to be rid of all of it, as the thought of having to have another sale was too painful. Watching people carry away my beautiful furniture, china, antiques, and patio furniture, as well as my Bose sound system and TV, even my expensive business suits and pumps, was humbling and horrifying.

One buyer asked if my speed skates were for sale. What had once been a prized possession was becoming extinct, being replaced by in-line skates. So many fond memories were held in those skates. I was the fastest backward speed skater at the rink. Every Friday night I lined up with six other speed skaters to race to the finish line for a twenty-five-cent Slushee.

"Okay," I said to the interested buyer, "ten dollars and they're yours."

Letting go of virtually everything was hard, but selling my twelve-string guitar was the toughest. I'd been writing songs and playing the guitar since I was eight years old. I'd taken private lessons from one of the best guitar players around, having heard him play at a fine restaurant while dining there with my father. He played guitar like Chet Atkins, and I was enthralled with his skill. My father inquired if he taught, and my first lesson was thus arranged.

My parents came to the first lesson. "Teach her to play the theme song to *Doctor Zhivago,*" my father requested.

"And teach her to play 'Amazing Grace,'" my mother insisted.

I eventually learned both pieces, but it was "Amazing Grace" that I was expected to play and sing at my parents' Christmas parties—certainly not my idea of fun. It didn't take my teacher long to discover that I could play by ear, which he remedied by switching the sheet music constantly to force me to sight-read. I practiced daily, until my fingertips would bleed, eventually forming calluses. Over the years my guitar became more than a musical instrument; it was a means of expressing what I felt inside. Selling it was not easy for me.

Fortunately, it didn't leave with a stranger. My best friend from high school bought it for her husband. Still, watching her carry it away, I felt as though yet another piece of my identity had been gouged out of my life.

When the estate sale was finally over and everyone had gone, I sat on the hardwood floor in my empty house and wept. Grief consumed me. Virtually all evidence of my former life was gone, and I was starting over with a dozen boxes of clothes and keepsakes. I had no idea of what to do, or where to go, or what the future held for me.

It was a great blessing to me that my friend Cindy, in Seattle, invited me to stay with her for a few months. She was retiring and wanted to show this Florida girl the great Northwest. I packed my camera, some warm clothes, and Alex and I boarded a flight. As we flew into Seattle, I saw the top of Mount Rainier, one of the highest elevations in the world, breaking through the clouds. Already the change of scenery was healing my broken spirit.

Cindy was a terrific tour guide. Our first adventure was driving up that mountain, past fields of tulips, cherry farms, majestic waterfalls, deer, wild ponies, and cute little chipmunks. As we continued up Mount Rainier the temperature began to drop dramatically. Snow covered the ground, and icicles hung from the walls of rocks that lined the road. We kept driving upward through white misty clouds until the sky cleared and we were able to look down. The view from above those clouds made me feel like a bird soaring to new heights.

The next morning we headed out to see Mount St. Helens. In 1980, sixteen years earlier, an earthquake had caused a volcanic eruption that had blown off part of the mountaintop, a sight that was seen as far as three states away, causing massive destruction of 230 square miles of thick, old-growth forest. The mudflows destroyed another 100 square miles of green growth. For more than a month following the eruption, the daytime sky was dark as ash continued to fall over the entire state and neighboring states.

As we approached the mountain, trees lay on their sides like thousands of scattered toothpicks. Riverbeds where water once rushed were now empty furrows, parched and cracked. Cindy drove to a nearby ridge where there was an overlook with a parking area, and we got out of the car. We walked to the edge and looked out over the devastation of the eruption site. All I could do was stare at the destruction, which went on for miles and miles, trying to comprehend the force of the blast that had caused such devastation.

As I gazed in silence at the barren land, covered with the carcasses of dead trees, I began to notice patches of green and new growth. Deep within the ruined landscape, seeds had survived the heat and the mud; they had made their way upward to the sun, sprouted, and now were growing. Seedlings of trees had taken root, filling in the spaces where their ancestors had proudly stood. In spite of the devastation, the land was still alive, and it gave off a very serene, spiritual energy.

As I breathed it all in, I recognized that my life was a lot like Mount St. Helens. We had both been tried by fire, and forced to find strength from deep within—strength to rise from the ashes.

After a few months of sightseeing, I was ready to return to Florida and resume therapy. My dad had invited me to live with him at his beach condo in Gulf Breeze, a beautiful island town near Pensacola, Florida. Fortunately, there was a well-known rehabilitation center just down the street. I had everything I owned—a dozen or so boxes of belongings and my car—shipped to his address, and I flew to Pensacola.

I loved my Nissan 300 ZX. When I had sold virtually all my belongings, I could no sooner have parted with my car than with my beloved cat, Alex. They were my pride and joy. I had bought the car from the original owner, who had garaged it and kept it in showroom condition. It had only twelve thousand miles on it and still had the original covers on the backseat. It was perfect. I kept it fourteen years while all my friends were driving either a BMW or a Mercedes-Benz.

"Think whatever you like," I'd chide them, "my car is beautiful and fast." My loyalty paid off when they became a collector's item after Nissan stopped making them in 1997.

Following the stroke, it was nearly impossible to work the clutch with my weak left leg, but I was determined to drive that car. Someone would have to pry my fingers off the gearshift

him to travel through northern Florida, he often stopped for a visit. Rhonna was another close friend who sustained me through that time. We had been close since high school, and she often wrote me letters that offered compassion, loyalty, and support. Over the years she never forgot my birthday and was always willing to lend a shoulder to cry on. There were other friends as well who helped me during that time. It was strange how the loss of friends who couldn't handle my disabilities just strengthened the bonds of friendship with those friends who remained true blue.

During one of Andy's visits we planned a day of canoeing on a river nestled within a rural area of the backwoods of lower Alabama. On the way, we stopped at a Stuckey's to buy some snacks. Near the cash register I noticed a fake Elvis driver's license and bought it as a gag gift for Andy.

It was a cool autumn day. The path of the shallow, crystal-clear water was framed by white sand dunes, and beyond them was a thick forest. It was so quiet that we could hear the wind blowing through the leaves. As Andy paddled, I photographed the sights. It felt good to be outdoors and behind the lens of my camera again. Except for an occasional deep spot, the river was shallow, and this was a comfort to me, as I was no longer able to swim.

At the end of the trip, as we turned the last bend in the deepest part of the river, the current suddenly picked up and we hit a log. Instantly the canoe overturned. Andy and I, and everything we had in the canoe, were dumped into the current. Stunned by the freezing cold water, clawing to keep afloat in my heavy clothes, I anxiously looked around for help. Unbelievably, two men were fishing on a nearby bank, just watching us. Suddenly I remembered my camera and reached into the camera bag that was still wrapped around me. My treasured Nikon and lenses had fallen into the river. Panic-stricken, I yelled to Andy. "My camera! Please get my camera!"

As soon as Andy made sure I was safely holding on to the capsized canoe, he dove deep for the camera. I looked up to see if the men on the shore were going to help us. Instead, they just watched us, entertained as they pointed at our belongings floating past them.

"Thar goes your hat," he said, pointing to the cap that Andy had been wearing that was now floating away on the current. Andy ignored his hat and dove back into the cold water again, this time resurfacing with the camera.

"The lens, Andy! Do you think you can find the lens?"

True friend that he is, Andy dove again and this time resurfaced with a triumphant look on his face, holding up my expensive lens. Once again I looked to the men on the shore and formed my cold, shivering lips into a call for help, but they didn't respond. They just continued to watch us, still pointing at our belongings floating past them. I clung to Andy as he swam me to shore where we climbed onto the bank, shivering, teeth chattering, clothes dripping, while the tobacco-chewing men continued to point at the amusing sight of our gear floating down the river.

Andy dragged the canoe to the rental rack, and we hurried to the truck, wet and cold, where Andy turned on the heater. All I could think about was my camera. I had to save it. It was almost five o'clock, and many of the small stores were closing.

"Andy, we have to get to a camera shop right away. I know where one is."

We arrived before closing time, and I rushed into the store.

"My camera's soaked!" I held it up to the elderly man behind the counter like a worried mother handing her sick child to a doctor. "Can you save it?"

Realizing the importance, the man offered to do his best and took the camera to his back room. Andy waited with me as we stood shivering, our wet clothes dripping on the old linoleum floor. Within thirty minutes the man returned from the back room.

"Your camera and lens are going to be fine," he said. "You got here just in time."

Back in the car, grateful we were okay, camera and all, Andy

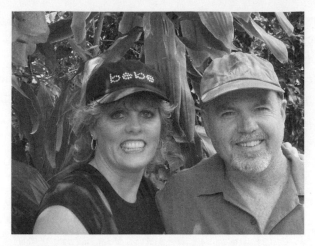

Andy and me

and I began to laugh about the incident. Suddenly I remembered the Elvis driver's license. I reached in the back pocket of
my still-wet jeans, but it was gone. It must have floated down
the river with our other stuff. I started laughing hysterically.

"What's so funny?" Andy asked.

It was several minutes before I could stop laughing long
enough to share the image in my mind of a couple of local fish-
ermen, like those men on the shore, who might someday find
that license floating by and shout, "Look, it's true! Elvis *is* alive!"

Though the eventful day had ended well, the experience of
nearly drowning made me realize that another loss had to be
regained. I needed more therapy so I could learn to swim again.

A year went by as I remained at my dad's beach condo
before returning to Orlando, where I began to see all the
rigorous therapies pay off. My speech was improving. My left
leg and left arm moved more fluidly. Even though I was still
self-conscious about my speech and my limp, I had come a
very long way. I was healing, physically and emotionally. I knew
that I would never return to my former life; instead, I held true
to my faith that there was a reason for my fate and that my
purpose was before me.

Critical Care for Caregivers

This, too, shall pass.

—Anonymous

STROKE SURVIVORS aren't the only ones who have to do a lot of letting go; so do their friends and family. In the beginning of the crisis they run on adrenaline, putting their own lives on hold without a thought. After the drama of life or death is over come the daily hospital visits, the long list of responsibilities to be shared, and so much to learn. After a while, friends and neighbors stop bringing over the casseroles. Then the phone stops ringing. Finally, the day may arrive when a caregiver can't remember the last time someone called and asked "What can I do to help?" Slowly reality sets in, and with it the necessity of shifting gears. It's time to prepare for the long haul and learn to let go.

The Loss of a Relationship

If someone dies, there's the finality of a funeral, when people acknowledge a loss and help the bereaved ones to express their grief. Unfortunately, there are no rituals for the loss of the person taken away by a stroke, and caregivers have difficulty finding an appropriate way to express their loss. Instead, they tend to mask their pain with a smiling face in order to be supportive around the survivor. They get so good at this facade that others often do not know how the caregiver really feels inside.

To compound their anguish and grief, very often stroke survivors are incapable of reaching out to physically touch their loved ones. Where in the past, smiles, hugs, kisses, and kind words would have conveyed the survivor's gratitude, caregivers must now be contented without demonstrations of thanksgiving or encouragement from their surviving loved ones. Caregiving can be a seemingly thankless job when survivors can't express their love and appreciation by word or touch. I often hear a caregiver lament, "If only he could hug me and tell me he loves me."

No one understands the enormity of loss in the aftermath better than someone who's been there, and I'd like to acknowledge it for you, the caregiver, in case no one else has done so: the one-on-one relationship you once had with a survivor has been drastically changed. It's no longer on the same footing. You feel as if your husband/wife/brother/sister/best friend has become your patient. Along with the other responsibilities you have assumed, you also must learn how to accomplish the delicate balancing act of protecting the safety of the survivor while at the same time maintaining the survivor's dignity and whatever is left of his or her autonomy. And all this needs to be accomplished rapidly, with little time to reflect on or plan how to provide better and more effective care.

A stroke is not like other diseases. When people recover from a heart attack or cancer, they are still treated like adults, but stroke survivors must relearn everything from the beginning— how to swallow, crawl, and communicate with words. Because they appear to be so needy and dependent, people tend to treat them like invalids. I can't describe the frustration this causes in survivors. No matter how they look on the outside, their feelings and thoughts are usually intact on the inside. But they are diminished when they are not respected as adult, thinking individuals.

On the inside I was still a clear-minded, functioning, mature adult who recently had been extremely independent and used to doing things in a certain way. Then suddenly I couldn't even speak. There were times when I just wanted to let go of my anger and scream out. *Leave me alone!* I wanted to scream. *Quit trying to cheer me up! Just let me sit here and be depressed. My whole life's been turned upside down. I can't walk, I can't talk, I can't even be myself anymore! Go away!*

Under such extreme circumstances, survivors can't help expressing their grief and loss in any way they can, even if it appears irrational. But in the wake of such a demonstration, caregivers often react by feeling even more guilty and responsible. How do you reason with someone who is being unreasonable? My suggestion is simple: don't try. Just ask them what they need. And if they want space, give them space, without personalizing their need as your fault.

Survivors often have emotional outbursts after physical therapy. Not only is it exhausting to get our bodies to move, we are exercising our brains as well, trying to get them to send signals to our muscles. In this jumbled, overloaded state we are capable of losing it over something as simple as having to a make a decision about what we want to eat or wear. It helps if our caregivers understand the source of this frustration. How to respond? Give them permission to vent their feelings. It is not personal!

But How about You?

Someone told me that she had asked this question of a caregiver who was overwhelmed with worry about her husband, a self-made man who had suffered a massive stroke and had to turn his thriving business over to his partner. Now he was home all day and angry all the time, bitter, despairing, and critical of everything she did for him. Was she doing too much? Should she give him more autonomy? She had been trying to convince him to see a psychotherapist, but he refused. At the end of her list of questions and concerns, my friend asked this distressed wife, "But what about you? How are you holding up?" The caregiver burst into tears. "No one ever asks me that," she replied.

Isolation and loneliness are often constant companions of a caregiver, but it doesn't need to be that way. If you're a caregiver, you are a member of a very large family, albeit clandestine at times. One out of five people in the United States is caring for an incapacitated loved one. Survivors of a massive stroke need the most care—an estimated forty hours a week. That's a full-time job! According to a study by the National Alliance for Caregiving, women account for 71 percent of those who work, full-time, at caring for a survivor. Of that group, of men as well as women, 88 percent had to quit their jobs or retire to meet their caregiving responsibilities.

These are monumental life changes. All caregivers in this situation desperately need someone who will help them meet the new challenges they face. I had to let go of a career, home, friends, and possessions, a series of profound losses that devastated me emotionally in ways I wasn't prepared to handle. Statistics show how many caregivers go through experiences similar to those of the survivors they care for. Unlike the losses we stroke survivors undergo, the sacrifices that caregivers make may not even be acknowledged. Caregivers must cope with profound changes in relationships within and outside their families; their very sense of self is shaken to the core as they relinquish long-held personal dreams and goals.

If you are a caregiver who has experienced these or similar losses, you are not alone. Other caregivers in this large family you belong to may be dealing with different diseases, but they have common concerns. If you don't have the kind of help that allows you time to go to a support group, there are all kinds of Web sites for people like you, and many of them have chat rooms. Thank God for the Internet!

One day I saw a sign with the familiar quotation "This, too, shall pass." I stared at it, trying to understand why it troubled me, and then I realized there was something missing: the words

"It's Not All Up to You"

Lotsa Helping Hands is a group of caregivers with a Web site and a chat room that also provides many links to other helpful sites. (You can find a long list of Web sites and groups for caregivers in the resources section at the back of this book.) Family Caregiving 101 is another group, and their motto is "It's not all up to you." That's a comforting thought, and it may not even have occurred to you! This group posted a list of ten commonly asked questions that address problems in the following areas:

1. Home care services
2. Web site support
3. Sharing responsibilities
4. Home care versus nursing home
5. Family relationships
6. Employers
7. Respite
8. Time management
9. Insurance
10. Finances

If you worry about any of these concerns, there are tens of thousands of people in a similar situation you can reach out to. They are waiting to help you feel less desperate and alone.

I would like to add another question to this list of concerns, one that caregivers need to ask themselves every night as they fall exhausted into bed: "What have I done for myself today, and what can I plan for myself tomorrow?"

"if you let it." Taking action makes all the difference. I have found that caregivers and survivors alike can become so immobilized by their circumstances that they don't know how to take the next step. But that *is* all they need to do. This, too, shall pass, if you let it.

8

In the Crucible of Change

———◆———

LETTING GO OF MY OLD LIFE was an enormous challenge, but not as daunting as the one I faced when I began to form a new life. The next five years were a true test of my character, my will, and my faith. Looking back on that time, I am awed that I found the courage to keep moving forward in spite of multiple losses and disappointments, with no hope in sight.

During the year following my stroke, friends within the medical and legal community urged that an investigation begin into the medical treatment I had received. Many questions remained unanswered: *Why had I not been started on a blood thinner sooner than thirty-six hours after my arrival in the emergency room? Why were my overwhelmingly obvious symptoms of a stroke overlooked? Why wouldn't anyone take me seriously when I insisted I was stroking?* Although I am opposed to frivolous lawsuits that plague our culture, I do believe that when mistakes are made, especially ones that cause severe injury, there must be accountability.

After lengthy consultations with medical and legal professionals and a lot of soul-searching, I decided to pursue litigation.

I knew that a lawsuit would be long and costly, and that I might
be disappointed in the outcome, but those factors didn't matter. My decision was based on principle. An injustice had taken
place; I was convinced of that. If I didn't take legal action, I
would be doing another injustice to myself.

Friends within the legal community began calling malpractice law firms, asking for support. Some firms replied that they
could not represent me due to conflicts; others came to my
home to hear my story. I quickly learned what I was up against:
only a few local firms had the resources to take on such a large
corporation. My situation became clear. It was like the story of
David and Goliath in the Bible, about a young boy who slays a
giant with only a slingshot. I felt like David standing before my
formidable foe. Night after night I lay awake, wondering if I
was doing the right thing. Should I just let go and leave the justice up to chance? But something inside me kept encouraging
me to keep going.

Finally, through a doctor I knew, I found lawyers who were
willing to review my case. Once again I told the story I had told
so often, and would repeat over and over again, about what
happened and didn't happen during the worst thirty-six hours
of my life. I was questioned for several hours, and they finally
agreed to take my case. For a while I was relieved, until they
informed me that it could take more than a year just to investigate and prepare my case—maybe longer. That would be an
excruciating test of my patience. Fortunately, I had had many
lessons in patience while recovering from my stroke. Although
I had no illusions about what lay ahead, I felt comforted to
have found lawyers who were in my corner and who would
bring my case to a just conclusion. Or so I hoped.

I put aside that worry to concentrate on my full-time therapy.
Every day I rode my stationary bike and walked on a treadmill.
At times I was so anxious to run I would increase the speed of
the treadmill when my therapist wasn't watching. To my disappointment, my left weak leg would buckle and I'd collapse.

For me, rehab was a safe haven where my limitations could be understood. I didn't feel different there. We had the privilege of asking one another questions that might be considered prying or even rude in the outside world. When it was my turn to share my experience, I'd explain how I had suffered a massive stroke at age thirty-one. The older patients would sigh and shake their heads, sad that I'd experienced such a horrific thing at such a young age.

I'll never forget the time I sat in the handicapped section at a professional baseball game. The entire row was filled mostly with elderly people in wheelchairs who looked at me and my friend in astonishment.

Why is she *sitting here?* I could almost hear them wondering.

I told my friend that I would be a minute, as I had some "politicking" to do. I leaned over and quietly said to a woman sitting next to me that I would love to sit closer to the ball field but because of my injury I was unable to manage the stairs.

"Well, honey, what *is* your injury?" she asked.

I explained that I'd survived a massive stroke a few years ago, and that at one time I was completely paralyzed on my entire left side. This launched her into reporter mode, and like wildfire, news of my condition spread quickly all the way down the row. Within minutes, strangers were asking me questions and sharing their survivor stories.

I turned back to my friend and smiled.

"Well, I'm in."

Times like this helped me to realize that I had been given a gift I had to share with others. After talking with so many survivors from all types of injuries and conditions, I could see that my experience inspired and touched lives. More importantly, it gave them hope. Sharing my story with the world became my motivation to keep getting better. Nearly every day I continued pecking with my one good hand at my keyboard, keeping track of my experiences.

. . .

Along with my rigorous physical therapy, I worked hard with my speech therapist, Terese. I was determined to speak and be heard above a whisper. Terese was the best! She was a one-of-a-kind therapist. Like so many therapists, she was kind and compassionate; what made Terese so special was that she genuinely cared about my future. She always encouraged me to one day become a motivational speaker, sharing my story of hope with other stroke survivors and leading the way in stroke recovery. Of course, at the time I thought this was absurd.

Nonetheless, I humored her. We would go outdoors, where the sounds of passing cars and the wind would muffle the weak sounds coming from my mouth. She would ask me to shout so she could hear me as she backed farther and farther away. At times it felt more like she was picking on me, but I now see that she was training me to project my voice. Speech therapy is so important in recovery, as speaking is our primary means of expression. And during the aftermath of a stroke is when I most needed to express myself.

I also sought out a number of alternative treatments as part of a regimen that is known as integrative medicine, incorporating treatments used around the globe, some of which have been successful for hundreds, even thousands, of years. These treatments included hyperbaric oxygen treatment (HBOT), cell therapy, acupuncture, reflexology, Eden Energy Medicine, Emotional Freedom Techniques (EFT), light therapy, cranial sacral therapy (CST), therapeutic massage, homeopathy, nutrition, and intercessory prayer. All of them were effective in my healing.

For the next couple of years, while I diligently continued doing everything possible to recover, I also was engrossed in my legal case. I found the work stimulating, and it helped me to focus on something other than word games, leg presses, and my next clinic appointment. Besides, I was eager to see the case through and have justice served. I had always enjoyed law but never imagined I'd find myself studying the process so intently. One of the younger lawyers working on my case became my mentor in the intricacies of malpractice law. He was tall, handsome, and extremely bright, and we quickly became friends.

I came to appreciate that although there appeared to me to be overwhelming evidence of negligence in my case resulting in damages, the challenge was proving causation. As the plaintiff, or the one bringing the matter to court, I had the burden of proof. As such, it was necessary to demonstrate that there was at least a 50 percent medical certainty that had I been started on a blood thinner when I arrived in the ER—instead of thirty-six hours later—it would have changed the outcome. Though common sense dictates that it most likely would have, I had to prove my argument with statistics and studies obtained from medical research. Unfortunately, since I was so much younger than most others who stroke, there were no comparable studies available, which rendered my claim particularly difficult to prove.

The legal process dragged on, year after year. For reasons far too complex to include here, I found myself changing counsel in midstream and feeling as though I had found my way into the Charles Dickens novel *Bleak House*, about a pitiful lawsuit that lasted decades and destroyed the lives of all the parties to it as it dragged on. Were it not so essential to my future, I would have washed my hands of it long before it was resolved. But some things are worth the wait, and everyone assured me that this would be one of those things.

To endure the frustration I felt during the long wait of my legal action, I scheduled a session with my psychologist, Dr. Anne Diebel, who had been a source of wisdom and support for me since my stroke. When I poured out the tale of my legal woes, she became greatly concerned that the intense stress could endanger my life by triggering another stroke. Eventually, however, Dr. Diebel not only helped me resolve my emotional distress, she also connected me to some of her legal friends, and it was through their help that I began to feel as though I would be sustained mentally and physically through the remainder of the lawsuit.

Though the legal process was arduous and anguishing, it was necessary. In my case, there were things that were awry in my medical treatment, and given the devastation of my stroke and recovery process, enduring the lawsuit was essential to guaranteeing that I would someday have a life to return to. My stroke had forced me to go through the anguish of letting go of the life I had planned. Surviving that experience gave me the strength to surmount multiple setbacks and painful losses in creating a new one. I did not realize then that the most difficult losses were yet before me.

I was no stranger to grief. In the turbulent household of my childhood, I had experienced loss. But I remain forever grateful for the calming influence of my grandmother. In the midst of my legal turmoil and my uphill battle to recover, I thought a lot about her and what she had taught me over the years. I was comforted by simply recalling her influence in my childhood.

When I was little, she would read to me as she rocked me to sleep. The book she read to me most often was from the Berenstain Bears series, the one in which the father bear gives his son a new bike. While the father demonstrates how to ride it, the little bear watches his father make many mistakes, barely escaping disaster. Each time, never admitting his obvious blunders, the father bear says, "Now, let that be a lesson to you." In the end, the little bear acknowledges his father as a great teacher who shows him what *not* to do. Little did I know then of the story's relevance in my own life, where the lessons of my childhood would prepare me for challenges I would face as an adult.

My grandmother saved this book in plastic wrap and gave it to me when I was in my twenties. By that time, I could see the deeper meaning of the story. We all come to learn our own lessons, but if we are wise, we can choose to learn from the experiences of others. I was blessed to have been taught so young that I could even learn from the mistakes of others. I keep this story book in a box of treasured memorabilia. I keep its lessons in my heart.

January passed, followed by a bleak, cold February, unusual for Florida. I should have recognized the ominous chill that blew across my soul when I received word that my grandmother had fallen. I rushed to the emergency room, where she had already been taken into surgery, and I paced the hallway with my mother and sisters. My grandmother was my best friend. *Did I have to lose her, too? Now?*

Finally, after three long hours, the doctor came out with good news. She was doing fine and would probably be able to start physical therapy the next day. But when I saw her, I could see how weak she was. Over the next few weeks she began to decline. The hospital staff did everything they could to help her, but she kept insisting that she just wanted to go "home." I knew what she meant, and I think she knew that it was too hard for me to accept that the "home" she wanted to go to was the one where she would be with her husband, my grandfather, who had died the previous year.

We made arrangements for full-time home care, and I went daily to visit her, finding her weaker each time. I was with her at the end. I held her hand as I felt the room fill with angels, giving me strength. I leaned over and stroked her brow.

"I love you," I whispered. "It's all right for you to go home. I'll be okay."

Moments later, she was gone.

My friends wondered how much more loss I could sustain. *How much loss can anyone take?* Until we have been tested in that crucible of change, we do not know what we can endure. Some people wither away, while others are tempered—emerging from those multiple losses stronger than ever. Had I never been in that fire, I would never have known how resilient I am, possessing the vitality to overcome whatever pain and suffering came my way. I was thrust into that crucible a victim, but I emerged a survivor.

Integrative Medicine

Conventional medicine specializes in treating the results.
We specialize in treating the causes.

—Mojka Renaud, L.N., Dipl. A.C.N.C.C.A.,
holistic practitioner

AFTER MY STROKE, I searched high and low for treatments that would help me recover, but I was disappointed in the results. Like millions of other Americans, out of desperation I returned to what used to be called alternative medicine. But that name no longer applies, because it's not an alternative anymore; it's going mainstream. Integrative medicine is a more accurate name, as these practitioners do not reject any form of medicine, conventional or otherwise, as long as it is safe and has been shown to work. It also integrates conventional medicine with healing practices that are used in the rest of the world, some of them for thousands of years.

According to Mojka Renaud, an acupuncture physician and homeopathic practitioner who has treated me for years, "Many clinical studies have been done on integrative medicine in Europe, but they have been suppressed in the United States. When I started practicing in this country twenty years ago, I had a difficult time collecting studies that were published here. Now they're commonplace. We're coming along, little by little."

Mojka grew up in Austria, where her father was a dentist. He died from mercury poisoning—he used mercury in dental fillings—and even though she was raised on organic food and didn't miss a single day of school, she also had high levels of mercury in her system. "In college I was studying foreign languages, but I developed mental problems. I couldn't remember any of the basic words in any of the languages, and it was very scary. That's what really drove me into natural medicine."

Finding the Causes of Health Problems

Metals and Toxins

Mercury, which is stored in fatty tissue, such as the brain, is one of the heavy metals that Mojka commonly finds in her patients. Studies show that a single microgram of mercury can damage neurons, but the mercury in a single filling releases 15 micrograms per day—the equivalent of eating 40 pounds of fish! Other metals and toxins that Mojka often finds in her patients are lead, which is stored in bones; aluminum, from canned food and deodorant; cadmium, in cigarette smoke and paints; fluoride, another neurotoxin; uranium, leached into soil near sites of phosphate mining; and arsenic, most likely from pesticides.

Environmental Causes

The number-one suspected cause of health problems in the United States is environmental. Mojka has been watching patterns for twenty years, observing more than five thousand patients over twenty thousand visits, and has discovered some very interesting links. She tracked down the source of E. coli in spinach to the manure of grain-fed cows. The intestines of grass-fed cows don't allow for the growth of E. coli. The same thing happens in a human body. The more pesticides that show up in her patients' tests, the more bacteria they show as well. The more heavy metals, the more viruses. High levels of heavy metal also can damage the arteries and blood vessels, especially the minute ones that deliver blood to the brain and other areas.

Holistic practitioners don't specialize in one area of the body. They have to know about every field because the body is a single organism; what affects one area will also have an effect on others. All these environmental toxins damage the immune system, and 85 percent of that immune system is in the intestines and the colon. When these organs are damaged by toxins the immune system breaks down, causing stroke and other degenerative diseases to develop.

Hypertension and Stress

A number of medical researchers report that stress is the underlying cause of 75 percent of all health problems. Therefore, stress and hypertension together constitute a formidable factor in the cause of a stroke. When people are stressed out they often say, "I just can't think right now." That's because stress increases the amount of cortisol produced in the adrenal glands, and raised cortisol levels restrict the flow of oxygen to the brain. It may explain why a lot of strokes happen on Mondays, holidays, and at times when people go through grief or major loss.

Cholesterol

Heavy metals, combined with adrenal exhaustion, are often found in people with high cholesterol levels. When the adrenals lose the ability to regulate cortisal levels, rising at night and falling in the morning, years of fluctuation will do damage to arteries already damaged by heavy metals and toxins that irritate the lining of the blood system. This causes inflammation, which the body corrects by walling it off with plaque.

Treating the Causes Holistically

The focus in integrative medicine is not treating cholesterol, for example, but eliminating the degenerative agents from the body and regulating cortisol production. That's why, instead of prescribing a drug that lowers cholesterol levels, holistic doctors treat whatever is causing the cholesterol buildup in the first place. This approach requires an understanding not only of cholesterol but also of the interconnectedness of all parts of the body and what it needs collectively to achieve balance and restore health.

Detoxifying the Body

A person can't go to the local vitamin store, buy some detox formulas, and flush out heavy metals and other toxins at home. In fact, this do-it-yourself method can be dangerous. People can become violently ill just from fasting. Detoxifying the blood can damage the kidneys, the body's environmental cleanup agency, when they become overwhelmed by a sudden onrush of toxins. A heavy-metal detox also puts a lot of stress on the heart. It can be damaged not only by the presence of the metals but also by detoxification *from* the metals.

Because of these potential dangers, it's really important to go to a qualified health practitioner who will perform tests to determine the types and amounts of toxins that are present in the body and prescribe a carefully controlled detoxification process. These testing devices have been used in Europe for fifty years, and they have finally been approved by the FDA for use in the United States. There are many kinds of modalities, such as electrodermal testing, that individualize the results and help doctors determine what a patient needs.

The preferred method of detoxification is the use of herbs combined with homeopathic medicines containing a sulfur compound, such as dimethylsulfoxide (DMSO) and methylsulfonylmethane (MSM). They are safe, gentle, and very effective in binding with metals and toxins for removal. They also don't overtax the heart and the kidneys. These compounds are used in combination with herbs and supplements, but they must be prescribed by a practitioner who knows what an individual needs and whether the ingredients are compatible. Foods containing sulfur are a natural detox. Some of them are eggs, cilantro, garlic, and certain types of algae (as long as they are not polluted; again, you might not be given that information at your local vitamin store).

Energy Medicine

We have entered an era where energy medicine is rapidly emerging into our health care system more powerfully than ever. Energy medicine is a well-documented science based upon the general premise that the body contains an invisible life force—a pattern of energy frequencies that can affect human health and promote healing.

According to Donna Eden, one of the foremost pioneers in this field, "The return of energy medicine is one of the most significant cultural developments of the day, for the return of energy medicine is a return to personal authority for health care, a return to the legacy of our ancestors in harmonizing with the forces of nature, and a return to practices that are natural, friendly, and familiar to body, mind, and soul." Energy medicine shows people how to prevent as well as treat illness. It is noninvasive and can be applied on a self-help basis.

Acupuncture

Acupuncturists say that application of needles stimulates neurons that are blocked and gets the electrical energy flowing again. In traditional Chinese medicine, energy is stimulated at points in the body called meridians to keep it moving and to restore balance. New technologies, such as low-frequency electro-stimulation acupuncture and electromagnetic biofeedback, have updated Chinese medicine in recent years.

Many recent controlled trials have shown good results in stroke patients who received acupuncture, especially in the acute phase or shortly afterward, and the most significant improvements were seen in patients who had the most neurological damage. The stroke patients who received acupuncture in these studies recovered faster than the control groups; had less pain and limb weakness; showed more improvement in speech, cognition, posture, finger dexterity, mobility, mood, and quality of life; and spent less time in hospitals and nursing homes—in one study, an estimated savings of $26,000 per patient!

Acupuncture for stroke patients includes manipulating the scalp as well as the body points, with or without electrical stimulation, and the sooner patients receive it, the better the results. Although emergency room physicians rarely know how to apply the treatment, some hospitals may have an acupuncturist on staff. It never hurts to ask, especially when the benefits of immediate treatment have been described in clinical studies as "strongly indicative."

Acupuncture, in combination with herbal medicine and physical therapy, also benefits patients who are treated within weeks, months, and even years after a stroke, with long-term results. In an ideal world, acupuncture would be a regular part of stroke treatment, from the emergency room to the rehab center.

Reflexology

The ancient healing art of reflexology utilizes a technique in which pressure is applied to specific points on the feet (and sometimes the hands) to promote relaxation and improve overall health. It is believed that the foot contains a coded map of the entire body and that particular points on the feet correspond to particular organs, glands, and body systems. Reflexology is another form of acupuncture, using fingers instead of needles to send an energy flow from the foot to the related organ. This technique encourages healthy functions in the corresponding areas of the body. The big toe, the reflex area of the foot that is related to the brain, is often sore or swollen in stroke patients.

Biofeedback

The use of electromagnetic devices that simulate the body's energy points is a technological update of the ancient form of energy medicine. The devices, which are accepted for use by the FDA, evaluate the conditions of body tissue, identifying them by light and sound as to whether an area is normal, inflamed, or diseased, and treating the area by adjusting the energy levels. It is used to treat stroke patients in ways that are similar to the treatment of acupuncture.

Color Laser Therapy

Each color has its own energy frequency, and by stimulating acupuncture points with various color lasers, practitioners can determine what kind of imbalance may exist in a corresponding organ and what is needed to treat it.

Nutrition

Blood clots, hypertension, high cholesterol, and stress are called the major causes of a stroke, but holistic practitioners do not treat them with prescription drugs and then treat their side effects with more drugs. They don't even call these conditions "causes." They call them "results" of a single factor: poor nutrition. The damage takes place on the cellular level. The outside of normal cells has negative charges that repel each other. Electrolytes such as potassium, magnesium, and the electrons in fresh, whole food help maintain the negative charge on the outside of the cells. Without these nutrients, the cells lose their negative charge and begin to stick together, forming clots.

Hemorrhagic strokes are attributed to high blood pressure that pops blood vessels, but the vessel walls have been weakened long before that happens. Once again, the real cause is poor nutrition that affects healthy cell repair and replacement.

Among the nutrients that will keep the walls of the blood system strong and the blood slippery are bioflavonoids, vitamin C, polyunsaturated fats, and essential fatty acids from sources such as flaxseed oil, primrose oil, and fish oil. Hydrogenated fats, on the other hand, have additives that cause the blood to clot.

Drugs prescribed for reducing cholesterol levels are known to block the production in the liver of coenzyme Q10, which helps keep the heart muscle pumping. Holistic practitioners lower cholesterol levels with diet and a heavy-metal detox. In one case, a man with congestive heart failure had been given five months to live by his doctors. His arteries were clogged with cholesterol, and the doctors had ruled out surgery. In desperation, the man found a homeopathic physician, who detoxified his system and treated him nutritionally. After a month, his cholesterol level had dropped by a hundred points. At his next checkup, his doctors were stunned.

Stress affects the amount of oxygen that reaches the brain by reducing the production of phosphatidyl serine and phosphatidyl choline in the adrenal glands. Holistic physicians prescribe these essential nutrients for the brain in powdered form, along with gingko and other nutrients.

Together with oxygen, glucose fuels the brain, which uses two-thirds of the glucose a person consumes. Sugar is a poor source of glucose, however, because it produces a quick spike in glucose levels followed by a quick drop. Then, when memory fades and people can't think straight, they tend to artificially raise glucose levels with another big dose of sugar, only to have it fall again. This rapid rise and fall of glucose also affects a person's ability to metabolize sugar and produce insulin, first becoming insulin-resistant and then developing diabetes, another major "cause" of stroke.

A better source of glucose for the brain is protein. A piece of cheese instead of a piece of cake will provide it a steady supply of fuel. Because blood sugar is usually low in the morning, protein is most needed at breakfast. Protein powders can be used for people on the run. Another healthy source of glucose is in fresh fruit, especially berries, ranging from blue to red to purple, because they also contain antioxidants, another important nutrient for the brain.

Living Food

We've always known that organically grown food contains fewer pesticides than inorganic food, but now we know that inorganic plants have 80 to 90 percent less phytonutrients than plants grown without pesticides. Plants produce phytonutrients to fight off insects and disease, but plants that have been sprayed with pesticides don't manufacture phytonutrients because there's no need. Phytonutrients in the human body also fight off disease, so when you eat them in organic foods, you are fortifying your immune system. This beneficial reason for eating fresh, whole, living food has only recently been discovered. There are undoubtedly many more reasons that remain unknown.

Food that has been processed or put in a microwave is sometimes called "dead" food because it no longer contains the living enzymes found in fresh food. In addition, any food that comes in a box or a can most likely contains potentially harmful additives, preservatives, or artificial flavors that have been added to make it more appealing and increase its shelf "life." If you can't pronounce items on the list of ingredients in a processed food, eating it may be a risk to your health.

Before the days of modern chemistry, when people grew their own food, everything was organic, and eating healthy was part of life. Temptations to eat unhealthy foods were few. Now eating healthy has become a choice, one that requires education and discipline. We've had to rediscover what our ancestors didn't even know they knew!

Eating healthy requires time, money, and effort, to say nothing of willpower, but together with holistic medicine, it is by far the best way not to have a stroke, or to prevent having another.

9

I Find My Voice

——◆——

MY RIGOROUS PHYSICAL THERAPY during these challenging years had resulted in my being able to walk fairly well, although I still had to use my cane. But my speech was still labored and weak, and I was frustrated over having made so little improvement. Then I had the good fortune to find Terese Uliano, who became my speech pathologist. She was the best— one of a kind! Like so many therapists who work with people with disabilities, she was kind and compassionate; what made Terese so special was that she genuinely cared about my future.

When I started working with her, my voice was barely above a whisper. I couldn't say much before I ran out of air, and what I did manage to say was still very slurred because I couldn't get my mouth to move so that it could form each word. I would joke with Terese about my slurred speech. When she first played back my tape-recorded voice, I said, "Gosh, I sound like a drunk. I was shocked and humiliated by what I heard.

Unlike stroke survivors who have aphasia or impaired cognition, my problem was dysarthria—neuromotor difficulty. I knew what people were saying, and I knew what I wanted to say, but I

185

couldn't get the words out. Imagine the frustration! I was locked out of the world of communication every bit as much as are survivors with impaired mental abilities, only in a different way. Although I was grateful I could walk again, I desperately needed to find my voice so I could express myself again, and I was determined to work hard with Terese to achieve that goal.

I had a big job ahead of me, as I had deficits in every area involved in speechmaking—motor difficulties in the mouth, diaphragm, throat, and chest that affected respiration, articulation, resonance, nasality, phonation, volume: the works. I expended so much energy in trying to speak that we had to schedule all my sessions in the morning, because by one or two o'clock in the afternoon I couldn't speak above a whisper. But Terese told me I wasn't starting from zero; all my hard work in physical therapy had given me a head start. The motor strength I had developed in other parts of my body would carry over into building up the motor strength I needed to improve my speech, and that encouraged me.

Terese provided me with strategies for improving each area of deficit, beginning with awareness. In the three years since my stroke, I had developed some bad habits I wasn't even aware of, such as my lack of respiratory support. When she had me try to blow a cotton ball across a table, I was amazed to discover that it barely moved. "See how little air you're using?" Terese said. "Without any air, you can't get your communication going." She explained that blowing on a cotton ball wasn't going to help develop my air flow, but it did help me recognize how little air support I was putting behind my words.

I was also unaware of how little I moved my mouth when I spoke. We sat beside each other in front of a mirror and she said, "We're going to say the same words together. Watch my mouth and then watch yours." Again I was shocked. I scarcely moved my mouth at all! I needed to become aware of how little I was using what I needed to improve my speech.

Another lack of awareness was the volume of my speech.

When I first listened to my voice on tape, it reminded me of
Marilyn Monroe's breathy whisper. She did it for effect, but I
didn't know I was doing it at all. I didn't even know *how* to
make my voice louder. It's something that people who can control the volume of their speech do unconsciously, according to
the environment they're in. When they go to a mall where
there's ambient noise or to a restaurant where people are talking next to them, they automatically talk louder, and it's not an
effort. For me it was, and I had to learn to do it consciously.

We began by working on respiratory support with exercises
that would help me use my muscles more efficiently. I was
amazed to learn how much good posture helped produce
speech. Stroke survivors have to learn how to sit up straight all
over again because the muscle weakness on one side of the
body pulls it down, putting strain on all the muscles. I had no
idea how much this affected my breathing until Terese asked
me to sit as if someone were pulling me up from the top of my
head by a string. "Take a deep breath and let it all out," she
said. Immediately I felt my torso expand and a slight increase
in the amount of air I could expel.

"Now crouch over, look at your knees, and take another
deep breath." I wasn't surprised when that posture decreased
the air I could take in, but when she told me to sit up straight
as I did before, visualizing that string pulling me up but this
time leaning to one side, I was amazed at how difficult it was to
take a deep breath from that position.

Once I was aware of how little I was using my muscles and
my breath, Terese gave me techniques that would help me use
them to the optimum. Running out of air wasn't simply a matter of the volume I took in; it also involved the rate at which
I had been allowing what little air I had to be expressed too
quickly when I spoke, resulting in that breathy kind of voice.
Terese told me, "When you're talking like that you're losing so
much of your vocal energy at the beginning that you're only
able to say a few words at a time. That's exhausting."

For three years I had been talking fast in order to speak as many words as I could before my breath ran out. Terese pointed out how counterproductive that was. Adding to low volume and slurred words, speaking quickly made me all the more difficult to understand, and it required even more energy when I then had to repeat myself. "People get tired of asking you to do that," Terese explained. "Unconsciously they just stop listening, and there goes the communication."

I had been unaware of how difficult it was to understand me. After three years of trying so hard to communicate, I simply didn't want to believe it. "I don't think I'm so hard to understand," I told Terese. Then she played one of our tapes.

"See why people are giving up?" I could tell by the look of compassion on her face that she knew how I felt.

"Don't be discouraged," she told me. "Look how much you've accomplished so far. You know what? One day you're going to share your story with other stroke survivors, and it's going to help them recover."

I thought this was absurd. Nevertheless, I humored her.

Terese gave me exercises in what she called vocal phonetory support, like taking a breath and silently counting as high as I could go before running out of air, and then counting backward. After I'd made progress doing that exercise, she said, "Good; now let's do it with speech." Once again, we did a lot of audiotaping to help me become aware of when I was losing my voice, because I kept insisting I wasn't. "What happened when you got to 'eight'?" she'd say.

"Okay, it died," I'd admit.

"That's when you need to take another breath. You just need to use it more efficiently."

Taking another breath may seem to be a ridiculously obvious solution, but for people with dysarthria, it's not. I began to realize that the reason for a lot of my speech problems was simply that I didn't know what wasn't working and why.

Speaking loudly can be a big problem, not only for stroke

survivors but also for people with Parkinson's disease and other degenerative disorders. When I tried to shout, I'd pull air into my lungs with all my might, force it out again, tighten up my vocal cords, and all that came out was a strangled, croaking sound. One solution for people who can't sustain their voice is a device called a vocal amplifier, but Terese didn't want to go that route with me. At times like this, she was great coming up with alternative techniques.

We went to a parking lot where the sounds of passing cars and the wind would muffle the weak sounds coming from my mouth. "Let's say you're in trouble," she said, "and your voice has to carry all the way across this parking lot." I took a deep breath and started shouting as she backed farther away from me. All that came out was a weak little "He-e-elp," like when you're try to shout in a bad dream and nothing comes out.

"Okay, let's try this," she said, holding up her palm like a traffic cop. "Imagine your voice has to hit my hand." Again she started walking backward. "Hit my hand!" she shouted. "Hit it!"

At times I felt like she was picking on me, but I now see that she was cheering me on, determined to find a way to use imagery that would get me to project my voice.

"Let's try this," she said one day in the parking lot. "Imagine you're standing on the beach. It's a beautiful day and the wind is blowing and the waves are coming in. Now open your mouth and try to grab as much of that fresh ocean air as you can."

That image truly helped. She was thrilled and so was I when I filled my lungs with that parking lot air and let out a blast. It wasn't exactly a shout, but it was close!

As my voice got stronger, she started calling me at about four o'clock in the afternoon. "Let me hear you," she'd say. At first my response was just above a whisper, but as the weeks went by I continued to progress until I could answer her with energy in my voice. One time she called me at six in the evening and I heard the usual "Let me hear you" at the other end of the phone.

"Can you hear me? How about now?" I replied, raising my voice. We both cried.

Terese also worked at a hospital as a speech therapist to patients in the rehab unit and in outpatient care. One morning when I came in for my session, I saw that she was not her usual enthusiastic self, and I said, "You seem off today." She replied, "I am, and I can't break patient confidentiality, but there's this young patient I just don't seem to be able to reach, no matter what I try."

The man was in his late thirties, and he had suffered a massive stroke resulting in a severe deficit in his cognitive abilities that had left him so depressed and angry that he had thrown his food trays at the nurses. He refused even to attempt to communicate with Terese. She was at her wits' end, the nurses were frustrated and dodging trays, and the patient was beside himself with his inability to communicate.

That morning Terese had tried to have a session with him, but he angrily kept repeating, "You—me—no—you—me—no." Terese told me she interpreted his words to mean, "You don't understand. You've never been here."

I listened to her intently, taking in her frustration. My mind was racing with thoughts and my heart was beating fast, but I kept quiet.

"And he's right, you know. I feel so ineffectual. How can I sit there and tell him what to do? I've never had a stroke. I just have to keep trying to find ways to get through to him."

"Let me talk to him," I said.

"What did you say?"

"Maybe he'll listen to me." Immediately I regretted my words. Who was I kidding? I still couldn't walk without my cane, and I stumbled over my words. I was no shining example of recovery. But it was too late. Terese was all smiles.

"You know what? You're right. I think that's a great idea."

I went into a long explanation of why it wasn't a great idea, but Terese wasn't listening.

"Let's try it," she said. "You can do this. I'm going to ask his family and doctor if you can come up and see him."

The moment I walked into that patient's room was life-changing. When he saw me—young, hobbling, supported by my cane—something changed in him, too. Meanwhile, Terese stood by, holding her breath. "Can I talk to you?" I asked. Immediately he recognized by my voice that I was another stroke survivor, and I think I felt that bond as strongly as he did.

He listened to me for about half an hour. I don't know if he could understand much of what I was saying, but that didn't matter. I was speaking his language, the one that only stroke survivors can comprehend. Although he didn't speak, I could feel I was having an impact on him, and he certainly was having one on me. I was doing okay in therapy, but motivation is the hardest part of recovery, especially after several years. While I was motivating him, he was motivating me. I had an obligation to recover that was bigger than myself. By the time I walked out of his room, I knew that my voice and my mission had found each other.

Afterward, Terese was so excited she couldn't stop talking. "I told you that you could do this!" she said. "I wish you could see yourself right now. It's like someone lit a fire in you! Think of how many people you can get across to that there's hope, Val! That they can't give up after the first twenty-four hours, or even the first few years. They just can't give up!"

After that visit, I hounded Terese for more exercises. Long ago I had made a promise to myself that if I ever got my voice back, I'd never stop talking about how I did it. I hadn't thought about that promise for years, because I didn't believe I ever would get it back. Now I felt differently. I knew I had a long way to go from walking into a hospital room to standing behind a microphone, but now I was on a mission.

And it's been like that ever since.

Strategies for Helping Survivors with Aphasia

If I were to lose all of my possessions save one, I would choose my speech, because with it I could regain all that I had lost.

—Daniel Boone, Ph.D., professor emeritus,
Department of Speech, Hearing Language,
and Science, University of Arizona

MOST STROKE SURVIVORS who lose their ability to comprehend suffer from aphasia. Although I had some aphasia, my communication problems were mostly neuromotor, a muscular weakness that followed my stroke. Though the source of our impairments may be different, all of us suffer from a sense of isolation, the pain of discrimination, and utter frustration. We feel isolated when people are impatient and fail to listen closely to our often indistinguishable speech; we feel discriminated against when we are dismissed as inebriated or unintelligent; and we feel frustration in the wake of the injustice of it all.

Although the work I did with my speech pathologist, Terese, focused on improving my motor function, I was most frustrated during my recovery when I was unable to express myself. Though I could usually write or scribble out words, I could not always verbalize the words I needed. Terese has provided me, for use in this book, with a number of techniques she uses for working with stroke patients struggling with the side effects of speech and memory limitations. I hope others will find these strategies as useful in helping to improve communication as they were in helping me. As you read further, you might think, "Oh, that's what my sister (or mother or cousin) is experiencing!" and, hopefully, you'll be better able to empathize with what she is going through and eventually be prepared to help bring her back into the conversations around the family table.

Word Retrieval

Stroke survivors with aphasia struggle with an inability to find words, and many give up and shut down. One woman suffered this impairment, though her other mental faculties were intact. She had always enjoyed her bridge club, but after a while, when she couldn't find a particular word, she would just quit talking. Out of frustration and embarrassment, she stopped going to her bridge club altogether and became increasingly isolated.

Caregivers and friends can help survivors who have difficulty with word retrieval. Not all words are inaccessible. If the elusive word is a thing, feel free to ask, "Tell me about it. What does it look like? What do you do with it?" If the word is a person's name, simply ask, "Tell me about her. What does she look like?" or "Is he a relative or a friend?" The objective is to keep the person with aphasia engaged in conversation. Eventually the listener may guess, "Oh, do you mean Joanne?"

"Yes! Joanne."

A connection has been made. It may not seem like progress, but neurologically these "Yes!" connections are also made in the brain. The survivor also receives the positive feedback of once again being part of the world of communication.

Sometimes people with aphasia can't retrieve a word but they can come up with the first letter. This strategy may seem to be like playing the game of twenty questions, but it works:

"Do you know the first letter?"

"It's a P."

"Paul?"

"No. Young girl."

"Oh, you're talking about Pat."

"Yes! Pat."

Once again, with a little help, the communication keeps rolling. The survivor may find that pointing to letters on a pocket letter board is helpful.

Another strategy is called topic maintenance. If the person suddenly goes blank and withdraws, you can say:

"You were talking about the play you saw last night."

"Oh, right."

A person with aphasia also becomes confused if the listener suddenly switches topics. It helps the stroke victim when the new topic is introduced by saying, "Now let's talk about your doctor."

"Oh?"

"When is your next appointment?"

Once her patient's confidence improved, Terese encouraged her to resume playing bridge with her friends and exhorted her to ask for their help. This she did, explaining to them, "Sometimes I can't think of words, but I'm going to start talking about this person or thing, and you might have to help me out." It's amazing how often survivors discover that family members and friends appreciate being able to help, even if they must assume some burden for keeping the conversation going. One of the woman's bridge playing friends told her, "I've missed talking to you. It's so good to have you back." Stroke survivors need to remember that they're not the only ones who feel isolated and disconnected. So do the people who care about them.

Slow, Small Sentences

Imagine that you have been sent to China, but you don't speak, read, write, or understand Chinese. Slowly you begin to pick up a few spoken words, although pronouncing them correctly is all but impossible. Even though you may know what these words mean in isolation, you're still in the dark when you hear the word used in a sentence.

Would hearing the words spoken louder help you understand their meaning? Not a bit. In fact, shouting would probably make things worse. Your problem is not hearing, and you haven't left your intelligence at home. You can't follow the conversation for the simple reason that you don't know the language.

That's how foreign their own language becomes for people who suffer aphasia after a stroke. They have difficulty with reading, writing, understanding, or speaking, with varying levels of deficit in each area. Some people may be able to understand more than they can read or write. Others may be able to read or write, but they can't retrieve words audibly. Some may regain all these skills quickly, while others may recover in a few areas but not in all.

Each survivor is unique. Generally, however, they all can benefit from being spoken to slowly, in a normal tone of voice (not as if they were children or had low IQs), and in simple sentences.

Watch for blank looks and silence, as they may indicate that your speech is too fast or your sentence structure is too complex for the survivor to follow. Keep your sentences short and simple, like you learned in school—subject, predicate, a few adjectives and adverbs—and speak slowly.

Telegraphic Speech

You also can take your cue from the way the stroke survivor speaks to you. One young man could understand what was being said to him, but he had lost the ability to read or write. His speech, however, was clear, but his access to words was limited. A conversation might go like this:

"What did you do over the weekend?"

"Oh, football, and see that game? Go, Panthers."

That's called telegraphic speech. With a little effort, his meaning is easy to put together by supplying the missing words: He watched the Panthers play football on TV; they won, and he's happy. People who judge his intellect based on verbal output would be surprised to know that he also could tell you each player's number, the position he played, and his stats. The young man was very knowledgeable about many subjects, but his verbal access to that information was limited. Although he's young, bright, and full of fun, he's isolated at school because people don't want to make the effort to communicate with him.

Gesturing

Some stroke survivors suffer a permanent loss of their ability to speak. Even they can learn to communicate, however, sometimes with such skill that as you watch them, you can "hear" what they can't say. This is not the same as sign language, which is limited to communicating with people who have learned to interpret that language. One man who had lost his voice found it through gesture. He learned to express himself that way so effectively that he could tell an entire story by pantomime and facial expression. What he couldn't get across by gesture, he drew. In the process, he discovered that he loved to draw and became an excellent graphic artist. Where there's a will, there's a way, and recovery may be filled with pleasant surprises.

Melodic Intonation

When I was in the hyperbaric oxygen chamber in the Dominican Republic, I discovered while watching *Terminator 2* in Spanish that it was easier for me to speak in that language than in English. Spanish, like Italian, is more melodic than English. Spanish consonants sound less precise and are not stressed as much.

Speaking Spanish also requires less breath than speaking English. Just ask opera singers what language they prefer to sing in—Spanish, Italian, English, or—the hardest of all—German, with all those long words and forceful consonants.

People who have lost their ability to speak have been known to still be able to sing. Because of these cases, the technique of melodic intonation has been used in speech therapy for years. Therapists try to find an intonation pattern that a patient can access and then put words on top of the intonation. For example, singing "We Wish You a Merry Christmas" becomes a singsong, "We wish you hello, how are you?" Unfortunately, the transfer from song to speech doesn't always bring results, but singing is fun. In Orlando, there's a group called Voices of Victory, which includes anyone who has had a stroke, including those with communicative disorders. While they can't speak, they can sing.

As Terese would say, "There are parts of your brain that still have words, so let's go find them."

10

From Powerless to Empowering

———◆———

IN APRIL 2001, my lawsuit was finally settled. For five years I had been repeating the story of my hospital experience over and over, each time taking pains to be as accurate and as factual as possible, and every time silently reliving those traumatic thirty-six hours. When I got the news of the settlement I felt as if that day was behind me at last. I could finally put it to rest and truly move on.

Everyone expected me to take off for a while after the lawsuit was resolved. But that was not what I wanted or needed. From 1996 until 2001, I felt as though I had been continually "away" from the life I had known before the stroke. Having to relive that crisis again and again only served to hold me back from reclaiming the ground I felt I had lost.

No; I didn't want to escape. I wanted to stay in the familiar here and now, in the city I loved, near the people I loved and who loved me. I needed to heal, not just my body, but also my soul. We all go through tough times in different ways. What I needed in the aftermath was to stay busy, and I did. I bought a new home and embarked on a remodeling adventure. I knew that home ownership would once again absorb my time or my money. In this instance, it required both.

Every day a fire needed to be put out, and as soon as it was, two more started up in its place. The budget I had set in the beginning went out the window about halfway through the project. Like a broken record, I kept hearing the words "Since you've done that, you might as well do this." Thankfully, my interior designer stepped in to save the day. With a few waves of his hand, the place seemed to magically come together. If I had never before realized the value of a professional, I did then.

By November my new house was completed, leaving me so exhausted that I felt as though I could have used a little remodeling myself. All I could do was "veg out" in front of the fireplace with my faithful friend and companion Alex. You can learn a lot about relaxing from cats. Alex would stretch out his furry, padded paws across the hardwood floor as he warmed himself by the fireplace, a sight sure to captivate anyone. I also spent the time with him reminiscing how far we had come together. It had been a long road with many unexpected twists and turns, but we had arrived at last—surrounded by all the creature comforts of our own home. We could now relax. I had even created a secret garden for him to enjoy. Every now and then I'd catch him chasing off an occasional drifter cat that had climbed our high garden wall to investigate what was behind it. Alex enjoyed being king over our domain once again.

Alex was by no means an average cat. Those who have bonded with their pets will attest to how animals become family members and take on many humanlike qualities (which some humans don't possess, such as Alex's ability to love me unconditionally, 24/7). I still can see him standing at the top of the stairs in those weeks after my discharge from the hospital. Alone and afraid, I would drag my left side up those dangerous open stairs. Alex, never taking his big, round eyes off me, silently assured me that I'd make it each time. I don't know what I would have done without him.

We had lived in our new home for six months when he became ill with kidney disease. Despite every effort to save him, his kidneys failed, and Alex died in my arms. He was an angel to the very end, even waiting until after I was settled in our new home before he moved on. In saying good-bye to him, I felt as if I had lost my best friend.

Everyone worried that I wouldn't be able to withstand so much grief and loss. As you would expect, my solution was to throw myself into several projects at once, to distract myself and to keep my focus off my loss. I knew I had to numb my pain. I couldn't stop moving the mountainous obstacles in my life; not now. I had accomplished too much.

In twelve-step recovery programs, people learn to take fearless inventories of their lives. For me, surveying my past served to strengthen my resolve as I was reminded of all I had achieved. I had gone from running a successful business to having a near-death experience. I had survived that—"made the cut," as Terese would say—and fired myself up to find out why I had been spared. I had started over and relearned how to walk and talk. I had lost my home, virtually all my belongings, and many friends. I had endured a long and fierce legal battle, and the deaths of my beloved grandmother and my cherished cat, Alex, all within a relatively short span of time.

Even so, I would endure yet more loss.

JULY 20, 2004

It was just another muggy day in July. My father was passing through Orlando on his way home from a business trip. Unbeknownst to my sisters and me, he had been experiencing chest pains the entire week during his business trip and had even struggled through an important presentation. But he put it out of his mind and focused on driving to visit his girls, only three hours away.

On the way, he phoned my older sister, Angie, and let her know he would be arriving shortly and wanted her to take him to the hospital, as he suspected he was having a heart attack. When he arrived, he maintained his calm and cool demeanor and even insisted on pumping gas into his SUV because he didn't want it to be on "E."

Thank goodness the hospital was only a few blocks away. Angie is very much like my father when it comes to remaining calm in a crisis. But I know her heart was pounding, and she was terrified. It was completely out of character for our father to ever want to go to a hospital.

When I received Angie's telephone call, she was clear that Dad was having a heart attack. I was in shock. Her words didn't register at first. Thankfully, a friend was visiting and drove me to the hospital.

Dad was in the emergency room and wired up to machines when I arrived. They said he had suffered a mild heart attack. I literally collapsed on his chest and wept. He placed his arm around me and began to cry with me. His chest shook. We both were scared.

The doctors told us they wanted to keep him for a few days before releasing him. Angie and I were pleased; Dad wasn't. He wanted to get back to his office and staff to deliver the big news about the account he had just secured. From his hospital bed he made calls on his cell phone to his partners, assuring them that he was fine and would see them in a few days.

One evening, as all three of his girls—Angela, Michelle, and I—sat in his room, we watched a video as he snacked on the green Jell-O that a nurse had delivered specially. The nurses were so charmed by his endearing wit and humor that they began calling him "Dan the Man." He even requested my black Ralph Lauren cap to wear because his hair was a fright. Dad always had to look good.

The next day he was transported to a larger hospital nearby that had the necessary diagnostic machines to properly assess his condition. The one-hour procedure turned into three as my mother and sisters, his girlfriend, and our pastor all paced the surgical waiting room.

Finally, the doctor came out walking alongside his gurney. Dad was wide awake and feeling fine. We were all relieved and thanked the doctor. As the doctor turned to leave, I glanced at him and thought I caught a hint of concern that went unnoticed by the others. I gave it minimal attention and ultimately let it go.

We all gathered around Dad's bed in his new room. I asked if he wanted anything.

"Yes, B, I'd love a Steak 'n' Shake burger. You know how I like it: mustard on one side, mayo on the other."

My friend and I dashed out to get a burger from Steak 'n' Shake, which, fortunately, was not far away. Upon my return, there were nurses in his room moving his bed up and down.

"What's going on? What's wrong?" I asked.

"It's my back—it's killing me, so they're trying to adjust the bed," he said.

"Okay. Well, let me put a pillow behind it and rub it. Where exactly does it hurt?" I asked.

We were all standing beside his bed when the heart monitor suddenly bellowed a haunting, flat-line beep. We all stared in stunned silence as Dad's hand went limp and nurses raced into the room. Down the hallway to ICU they rushed him. Running behind his gurney I yelled, "Dad, I'm right behind you! Hang on!"

I was a crazy woman. While the others stood obediently outside the door to the isolated room, I barged in and screamed, *"DAD!"*

Within seconds I was removed from the room, but not fast enough for me to avoid seeing the doctors pounding on his chest, trying to revive him. I was given something to calm me, and I fell into a trance. I hung on to a railing and began to pray, begging God not to let him go. But Dad was already gone. Even so, the doctors kept him artificially alive, hoping he would come back. All night we waited, and in the early morning hours we were allowed to see him.

My sisters, my mother, his girlfriend, and I were taken to a room where he laid, eyes closed, his heart being pumped by a machine. Dad was gone. We knew it. I even felt his spirit comforting me that he was not in that body; he was free. The doctor explained that we needed to make our decision. As we each took turns saying our good-byes, I lay my head on his chest and wept.

On Friday, July 23, 2004, he was buried. The marines fired a gun salute and played "Taps" as a crate of white doves were set free.

The following months were a blur. I was completely spent, once again tried beyond what I thought I could bear. But I was wrong—I was to be even further challenged as I faced down the infamous four major hurricanes that hit Florida from August to November that year. So consumed by grief for the loss of my father, I never left my home to seek safety. I just wanted to die so I could be with my daddy.

When silver is being refined, a fire blazes beneath the crucible as the silversmith stirs the precious metal until dross begins to appear at the surface. The silversmith patiently skims the surface of the silver, removing the dross, and then continues to stir up the pot again and again, each time removing the dross that surfaces. He knows the process is complete when he is finally able to see his own reflection in the surface of the heated silver. Without having been stirred up, however, the silver would remain imperfect, flawed and devalued.

My fiery journey of loss, suffering, and change served to stir up my life in much the same way. In the refining process I learned many valuable lessons that will carry me forward throughout my life. We are not in control of our lives, but we *can* decide how we will respond to our circumstances. Each of us will face challenges and obstacles in this life and, depending on how we navigate them, we can be blessed with a multitude of gifts and talents that can be gleaned from those experiences. We can choose to allow our trials to become our testimonies.

During my long and arduous struggle to recover, I found that even a stroke has purpose and can be useful. In fact, in my life, my stroke stretched me in ways I could never have imagined. I discovered that many answers I had sought to the questions of life were already within me. On my journey, I encountered what had been inside of me all along: the fire within my soul.

My miraculous recovery has proved that faith does move mountains. Learning to walk again taught me that nothing is impossible. The loss of loved ones taught me that life does end, and to spend time with those you love as much as you can while they're with us. Overcoming a fierce lawsuit taught me that justice can prevail against all odds, even for a pint-sized David against a towering and powerful Goliath. My many challenges taught me to let go and trust. All I had to do was show up and do the next right thing.

Would I wish what I went through on anyone else? Never. Do I regret that it happened? No, because it has purpose and is useful to help others. Sometimes I joke about it by saying, "If I hadn't had my stroke I'd be just another estate planner. Now look at me." It's a gift to be able to travel the country, inspiring all those stroke survivors in ways no doctor ever can, because I've been where they've been, suffered the way they've suffered, and still made it through.

My experiences prepared me for public speaking. When I was getting ready to make my first speech, I was naturally scared and filled with butterflies. I had prepared an outline and even had the event coordinator help me write it so I would be sure to cover all the important points. I couldn't help wondering, however, why people would want to listen to *me*. I also was very self-conscious of my speech impairment, fearing that my audience might not be able to understand me.

I shared my concerns with the coordinator, who assured me, "Experts can talk about facts and figures all day long, but your audience wants to hear from a survivor."

"You're a messenger," she added. "Don't forget that, and you'll be fine."

Her words were exactly what I needed to hear.

When I walked onto that stage to give my first speech, I saw a room full of people, many of them in wheelchairs, slumped to one side the way I used to be, people who couldn't talk but desperately wanted to, people who were imprisoned inside their bodies but wanted to get out. Instantly my heart opened up to them. I forgot all my fears and began to speak. After a

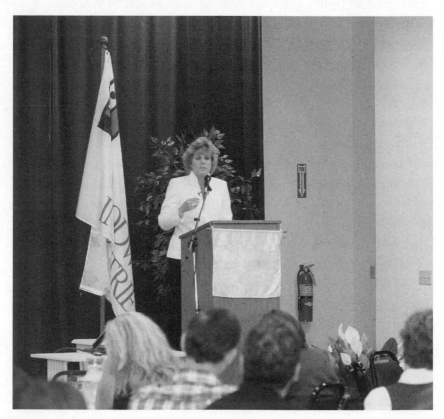

Giving a speech

while I was so into the flow of my thoughts that I realized I wasn't following my outline. I paused, embarrassed, frantically scanning my notes, then said to the waiting audience, "I have no clue where I'm at." That got a good laugh, and I started laughing as well. I didn't use the notes after that, but just spoke from my heart. I became a vessel. The message went into me and out to them.

My story has encouraged so many people, and it's become my mission to reach as many as I can. That's why I've written this book. In the process I found out much more about strokes than I ever thought possible, with more to be learned every day. I also found out that one of the most dangerous risk factors for a brain attack is the incredible amount of ignorance about this catastrophe that strikes millions of people and accounts for more disability than any other disease. I was amazed to read a recent survey that found that one out of three people do not know even the most obvious symptoms of a stroke. I hope that this book, as part of a rapidly growing campaign of stroke awareness, will help to change that alarming statistic.

All the recent discoveries about the brain are also helping to increase awareness about strokes. When there's an exciting development, it makes the news. Now there are television programs and magazine articles about this disease as there never have been before. Because of the expedient response time that has been implemented by the hospital where I had my stroke, many lives have been saved. We all make mistakes, and we grow when we learn from them. I honor the hospital where my stroke happened for its current expanded expertise in stroke awareness, detection, and treatment.

To solve a problem, especially one with the magnitude of stroke, we must first become aware of it. Thankfully, that is beginning to happen. It's why I devote my time to speaking out about the national epidemic of strokes that is killing or disabling our friends, parents, sisters, brothers, aunts, uncles,

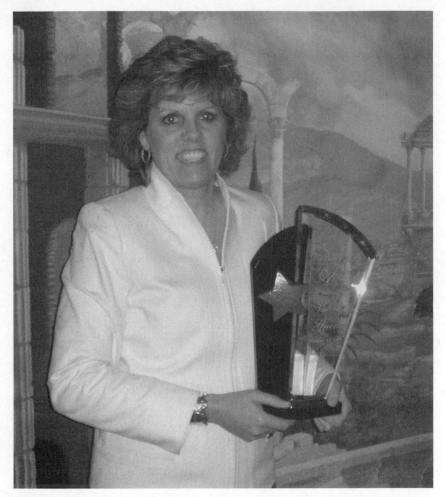

Receiving a Celebration of Life award

grandparents—even children and babies. My goal is to educate
and raise awareness not only about the problem of stroke but
also about its solutions.

If enough people know the warning signs of a stroke, and
know that it can happen to any of us—anywhere—that awareness alone will save countless lives. If we see someone in a
mall, restaurant, or theater exhibiting signs of a stroke, we will
not jump to the conclusion that the person is inebriated or on

drugs but know that person needs to get to an emergency room as soon as possible. If a friend tells us of an incident of extreme dizziness or sudden slurred speech for no reason, we'll know that we must urge that person to make an appointment with a neurologist or stroke specialist right away.

If enough of us hold a collective intention to find solutions to strokes, new effective prevention and treatment options will become available. Many powerful methods have been described in this book, and many more are in the pipeline. But as one neurologist put it, "The best way to treat a stroke is not to have one." That's not as cynical as it sounds. For the most part, a stroke is a preventable disease. Nearly all the risk factors can be treated or avoided.

Because of all the recent breakthroughs, many people in the field of stroke medicine are calling this the decade of the brain. It's time to give this priceless, irreplaceable part of our body the attention it deserves. We can all start by doing everything possible to keep a stroke from happening.

I am a woman with a mission. I am carrying this message to as many who will listen in the hopes of saving lives. It is a sacred privilege and moves me deeply to see the faces of my fellow stroke survivors light up when I walk into a hospital room or speak to a group. Looking at me, they realize there is hope. My having been where they are speaks volumes to them. When someone in a wheelchair takes my hand and sobs, "I was the head of my company, and look at me now," I am filled with compassion. I stand, unassisted, look them square in the eye, and speak my message into their heart:

"I know where you're at. I was the head of a company, too. I was in a wheelchair just like you, drooling, face drooping, unable to speak, filled with anguish and despair. But look at me now!"

EPILOGUE

Giant Leaps Ahead

———◆———

THE BRAIN IS THE LAST FRONTIER. We know about stars that are lightyears away, and we know about the smallest microbe, but the brain has remained a mystery—until now. In the past decade, the development of new technology, which has always led the way in unlocking the secrets of the universe, has now given us the power to unlock the secrets of the very thing that makes us human.

During the decade of the brain, which began in 1996 with the FDA's approval of tPA, the statistics for stroke mortality fell, while at the same time the age of the population rose. That's a beginning. During that time as well, the concept of the recoverable brain opened up an entire continent of new research that has resulted in a revolutionary approach to stroke treatment and recovery. This first good news ever about strokes broke through the media's wall of silence at last, and stroke awareness is increasing. People are finally paying attention to the need to take care of their brains. The future looks truly promising for every aspect of stroke medicine—prevention, treatment, and recovery.

It's an exciting time to be alive! A revolution in health care is taking place as we become aware of ways to treat and prevent illnesses more effectively. The following are just two promising examples of things to come.

Diagnosing and Predicting Stroke

What makes a stroke so dangerous is the way it sneaks up on you. The dilemma has always been trying to find a diagnostic test that will predict a stroke.

Such a test already exists in Europe and is in the process of being approved for clinical trials in the United States. It identifies the presence of a subtype of a glutamate receptor called NR2 peptide and its antibodies, which are brain-related disease markers predicting an onset of an ischemic stroke. Such a test, called Gold Dot, is being used at a dozen hospitals in the United States, and plans are being made for extended multicenter clinical trials.

Stem Cell Research

Live cell therapy has been available in Europe since the 1940s, when Paul Niehans, a Swiss physician, developed a treatment that employed injecting live cells from a sheep embryo into patients at La Prairie, a famous clinic where celebrities and heads of state still go to be rejuvenated and treated for illness. This treatment has never been accepted by the medical establishment in the United States, where it is viewed as an extreme and dangerous form of quackery. Yet politicians and the media in the United States continue to define human embryonic stem cells as pioneering and most promising, all the while ignoring the incredibly lengthy body of evidence attesting to the success of alternative sources for cells!

In combination with hyperbaric oxygen therapy (HBOT),

which I still receive today, I credit live cell therapy as attributing to my amazing recovery. Although a number of states have passed medical access laws for live cell therapy that protect doctors on a state level, physicians in the United States who treat patients with this therapy usually do not advertise it. The most common way they meet patients is by word of mouth, and that situation is not likely to change. Nevertheless, recent stem cell researchers have confirmed what Niehans said all along: embryonic stem cells can grow into any cell in the body, where they wrap themselves around existing damaged cells, rejuvenate, and replicate them.

As this book goes to press, two teams of scientists have successfully reprogrammed human skin cells into stem cells, "blank slates" that act like embryonic stems cells in their ability to grow into any other type of cell in the body. Not only does the use of human skin cells bypass the religious and ethical objections of the use of human embryos that have delayed the progress of stem cell research for years, particularly in the United States, it also provides a genetic match for the patient. Stem cell researchers have called this news "electrifying," and the race is on in laboratories around the world to develop the use of human skin cells in the treatment of stroke, cancer, Alzheimer's, and a host of other diseases that plague our world.

Improvements in diagnosis and treatment are but two examples of the explosion of research that is causing so much excitement in stroke medicine. The future will undoubtedly bring many more. These new inroads are sources of great comfort and encouragement to me and, I hope, to each of you reading my story.

Parting Thoughts

In May 2007, my sisters and my mother gathered at *my* house for a Mother's Day celebration. It was glorious to be alive, to

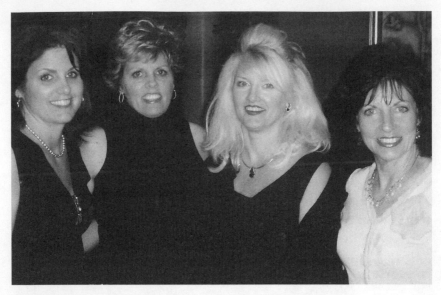

Michelle, me, Angie, and Mom

cook and decorate and host my family in my own home. I have been restored not only physically but also emotionally and even spiritually. It was a crowning moment, a just dessert for having worked very long and very hard.

The fire within me that drove me to persevere for my own recovery continues to motivate me today as I reach out to other stroke victims and caregivers. My goal is to educate and raise awareness about both the problem of strokes and their solutions so that this next generation will ask, "What's a stroke?" in the same manner that my generation asks, "What's polio?" If enough of us know the warning signs of a stroke, and know it can happen to any of us, anywhere, countless lives will be saved.

If I can help make that happen, I will not have suffered in vain.

With love and light,
Valerie

Resources

I compiled the following directories of hospitals and rehabilitation centers by searching through Web sites on the Internet. Although these lists are by no means complete, they are by far the most comprehensive to date. Including these facilities is not an advertisement or a recommendation; it is a service I am glad to provide to stroke patients and their families, because I know this information will save lives and help people heal from the ravages of a stroke.

Acute Care

This state-by-state guide to more than 650 designated stroke centers is a combination of lists that can be found on the Web sites of the American Heart Association and the American Stroke Association, the National Stroke Association, the certification program of the Joint Commission for Accreditation of Healthcare Organizations (JCAHO), and information provided on the Web sites of a number of state departments of health. As many hospitals are currently working toward becoming accredited stroke centers, I recommend going to their Web sites (see "Stroke Organizations" on page 246 and "Organizations for Caregivers" on page 247).

Hospitals with Stroke Centers
An asterisk following the name of a hospital in the following list indicates that that hospital assists community hospitals by telephone in treating acute stroke. A dagger indicates that the hospital receives this service. If you do not live near a stroke center, contact your local hospital and ask whether it is connected to an outreach program.

ALABAMA

Decatur General Hospital
Decatur, AL

South Baldwin Regional Medical
   Center
Foley, AL

University of South Alabama
   Medical Center
Mobile, AL

ALASKA

Alaska Regional Hospital*
Anchorage, AK

The Rural Hospital Flexibility
   Program provides service to this
   vast and mostly rural state. For
   details call (907) 465-8618
   (Juneau) or (907) 269-3456
   (Anchorage)

ARIZONA

Barrow Neurological Institute of
   St. Joseph's Hospital*
Services forty-three outlying
   hospitals
Phoenix, AZ

Condelet St. Mary's Hospital
Tucson, AZ

Mayo Clinic Hospital
Phoenix, AZ

Sparks Regional Medical Center
Fort Smith, AZ

Verde Valley Medical Center
Cottonwood, AZ

ARKANSAS

St. Vincent Hospital
Little Rock, AR

CALIFORNIA

Brotman Medical Center
Culver City, CA

California Pacific Medical Center
San Francisco, CA

Cedars-Sinai Medical Center
West Hollywood, CA

CHW Dominican Hospital
Santa Cruz, CA

Doctors Hospital of Manteca
Manteca, CA

Doctors Medical Center of
   Modesto
Modesto, CA

El Camino Hospital
Mountain View, CA

Fountain Valley Regional Hospital
   and Medical Center
Fountain Valley, CA

Glendale Adventist Medical
   Center
Glendale, CA

Good Samaritan Hospital (San
   Jose)
San Jose, CA

Hoag Memorial Hospital
Newport Beach, CA

John Muir Medical Center
Concord Campus
Concord, CA

John Muir Medical Center
Walnut Creek Campus
Walnut Creek, CA

Kaiser Foundation Hospital
Santa Clara Medical Center
Santa Clara, CA

Kaiser Foundation Hospital
Redwood City
Redwood City, CA

Kaiser Foundation Hospital
Sacramento/Roseville
Sacramento, CA

Kaiser Foundation Hospital
Santa Teresa
San Jose, CA

Mercy General Hospital
Sacramento, CA

Mercy San Juan Medical Center
Carmichael, CA

Mills-Peninsula Health Services
Burlingame, CA

Mission Hospital Regional Medical
   Center
Mission Viejo, CA

O'Connor Hospital
San Jose, CA

Palomar Medical Center
Escondido, CA

Pomerado Hospital
Poway, CA

Salinas Valley Memorial
   Healthcare System
Salinas, CA

San Diego Medical Center
San Diego, CA

Scripps Memorial Hospital,
   Encinitas
Encinitas, CA

Sharp Grossmont Hospital
La Mesa, CA

Sharp Memorial Hospital
San Diego, CA

Shasta Regional Medical Center
Redding, CA

Sierra Vista Regional Medical
   Center
San Luis Obispo, CA

Stanford Hospital and Clinics
Stanford, CA

Sutter Medical Center, Sacramento
Sacramento, CA

UCLA Medical Center
Los Angeles, CA

UCSF Medical Center
San Francisco, CA

University of California
Irvine Medical Center
Orange, CA

University of California
San Diego Medical Center
San Diego, CA

Valley Care Medical Center
Pleasanton, CA

Woodland Healthcare
Woodland, CA

COLORADO

Centura Health/Littleton Adventist
   Hospital
Littleton, CO

Centura Health/St. Anthony
   Hospital
Denver, CO

Denver Health Medical Center
Denver, CO

Health One/Presbyterian St. Luke's
   Medical Center
Denver, CO

Memorial Hospital
Colorado Springs, CO

North Suburban Medical Center
Thornton, CO

Parkview Medical Center
Pueblo, CO

Presbyterian/St. Luke's Medical
   Center
Denver, CO

St. Anthony Central Hospital
Denver, CO

St. Mary Corwin Medical Center
Pueblo, CO

Swedish Medical Center
Colorado Neurological Institute
Englewood, CO

CONNECTICUT

Danbury Hospital
Danbury, CT

Greenwich Hospital
Greenwich, CT

Hartford Hospital
Hartford, CT

Middlesex Hospital
Middletown, CT

Norwalk Hospital
Norwalk, CT

St. Vincent's Medical Center
Bridgeport, CT

Yale–New Haven Hospital
New Haven, CT

DELAWARE

Beebe Medical Center
Lewes, DE

DISTRICT OF COLUMBIA

George Washington Hospital
   Center
Washington, DC

FLORIDA

Baptist Hospital
Pensacola, FL

Bay Medical Center
Panama City, FL

Bayfront Medical Center
St. Petersburg, FL

Bethesda Memorial Hospital
Boynton Beach, FL

Blake Medical Center
Bradenton, FL

Cape Canaveral Hospital
Cocoa Beach, FL

Central Florida Regional Hospital
Sanford, FL

Charlotte Regional Medical Center
Punta Gorda, FL

Cleveland Clinic Hospital
Weston, FL

Community Hospital
New Port Richey, FL

Delray Medical Center
Delray Beach, FL

Doctor P. Phillips Hospital
Orlando, FL

Doctors Hospital of Sarasota
Sarasota, FL

Edward White Hospital
Saint Petersburg, FL

Fawcett Memorial Hospital
Port Charlotte, FL

Florida Hospital, Altamonte
Altamonte Springs, FL

Florida Hospital, Deland
Deland, FL

Florida Hospital, Flagler
Palm Coast, FL

Florida Hospital, Orlando
Orlando, FL

Florida Hospital, Ormond
   Memorial
Ormond Beach, FL

Florida Medical Center
Lauderdale Lakes, FL

Good Samaritan Medical Center
West Palm Beach, FL

Gulf Coast Medical Center
Panama City, FL

Halifax Medical Center
Daytona Beach, FL

Hialeah Hospital
Hialeah, FL

Holmes Regional Medical Center
Melbourne, FL

Holy Cross Hospital Ministries
Fort Lauderdale, FL

Indian River Memorial Hospital
Vero Beach, FL

JFK Medical Center
Atlantis, FL

Lakeland Regional Medical Center
Lakeland, FL

Lakewood Ranch Medical Center
Bradenton, FL

Largo Medical Center
Largo, FL

Lawnwood Regional Medical
    Center
Lawnwood, FL

Leesburg Regional Medical Center
Leesburg, FL

Manatee Memorial Hospital
East Bradenton, FL

Mayo Clinic/St. Luke's Hospital
Jacksonville, FL

Mease Countryside Hospital
Safety Harbor, FL

Mease Dunedin
Dunedin, FL

Memorial Hospital West
Pembroke Pines, FL

Memorial Regional Hospital
Hollywood, FL

Morton Plant Hospital
Clearwater, FL

Morton Plant North Bay Hospital
Dunedin, FL

Morton Plant North Bay Hospital
New Port Richey, FL

Munroe Regional Medical Center
Ocala, FL

North Broward Medical Center
Deerfield Beach, FL

Northside Hospital
St. Petersburg, FL

Oak Hill Hospital
Brooksville, FL

Orlando Regional Medical Center
Orlando, FL

Orlando Regional Sand Lake
    Hospital
Orlando, FL

Palm Bay Community Hospital
Palm Bay, FL

Palm Beach Gardens Medical
    Center
Palm Beach Gardens, FL

Palms of Pasadena Hospital
St. Petersburg, FL

Parrish Medical Center
Titusville, FL

Peace River Regional Medical
    Center
Charlotte, FL

Pinecrest Rehabilitation Hospital
DelRay Beach, FL

Regional Medical Center
Bayonet Point
Hudson, FL

Sacred Heart Health System
Pensacola, FL

St. Anthony's Hospital
St. Petersburg, FL

St. Joseph's Hospital
Tampa, FL

St. Lucie Medical Center
Port Saint Lucie, FL

Sarasota Memorial Hospital
Sarasota, FL

Seven Rivers Regional Medical
    Center
Crystal River, FL

Southwest Florida Regional
    Medical Center
Fort Myers, FL

Tallahassee Memorial Regional
Tallahassee, FL

Tampa General Hospital
Tampa, FL

University of Florida
Shands-Jacksonville Medical
    Center*
Provides assistance and helicopter
    transport to rural northeastern
    Florida
Jacksonville, FL

West Boca Medical Center
Boca Raton, FL

West Florida Regional Medical
    Center
Pensacola, FL

Westside Regional Medical Center
Plantation, FL

Winter Haven Hospital
Winter Haven, FL

Wuesthoff Medical Center
Melbourne, FL

Wuesthoff Medical Center
Rockledge, FL

GEORGIA

Atlanta Medical Center
Atlanta, GA

DeKalb Medical Center
Decatur, GA

Doctors Hospital of Augusta
Augusta, GA

Emory University Hospital
Atlanta, GA

Floyd Healthcare Management
Rome, GA

Grady Health System
Atlanta, GA

Gwinnett Medical Center
Lawrenceville, GA

Habersham County Medical
    Center
Demorest, GA

Hamilton Medical Center
Dalton, GA

Medical Center of Central Georgia
Macon, GA

Medical College of Georgia Health
Augusta, GA

Memorial Health University
    Medical Center
Savannah, GA

North Fulton Medical Center
Roswell, GA

Piedmont Hospital
Atlanta, GA

St. Francis Hospital
Columbus, GA

St. Joseph's/Candler Health System
Savannah, GA

St. Mary's Health Care System
Athens, GA

HAWAII

Castle Medical Center
Kailua, HI

Kaiser Permanente Hawaii
Honolulu, HI

Kapi'olani Medical Center at Pali
Momi
Aiea, HI

North Hawaii Community Hospital
Kamuela, HI

Queens Medical Center
Honolulu, HI

ILLINOIS

Advocate Christ Medical Center
Oak Lawn, IL

Advocate Good Samaritan
Hospital
Downers Grove, IL

Advocate Health Care
Oak Brook, IL

Advocate Lutheran General
Hospital
Park Ridge, IL

Alexian Brothers Medical Center
Elk Grove Village, IL

Blessing Hospital
Quincy, IL

Edward Hospital and Health
Services
Naperville, IL

Evanston Northwestern
Healthcare
Evanston, IL

Loyola University Medical Center
Maywood, IL

Mercy Hospital and Medical Center
Chicago, IL

Methodist Medical Center of
Illinois
Peoria, IL

Northwestern Memorial Hospital
Chicago, IL

OSF Saint Francis Medical Center
Peoria, IL

Rush Medical Center
Chicago, IL

Sherman Hospital
Elgin, IL

St. Alexius Medical Center
Hoffman Estates, IL

Swedish American Hospital
Rockford, IL

University of Illinois
Medical Center at Chicago
Chicago, IL

INDIANA

Bloomington Hospital
Bloomington, IN

Bluffton Regional Medical Center
Bluffton, IN

Clarian Health Partners
Indianapolis, IN

Columbus Regional Hospital
Columbus, IN

Deaconess Hospital
Evansville, IN

Lutheran Hospital of Indiana
Fort Wayne, IN

Parkview Hospital
Fort Wayne, IN

St. Joseph Regional Medical Center
South Bend, IN

St. Mary's Medical Center
Evansville
Evansville, IN

St. Vincent Hospitals and Health
Services
Indianapolis, IN

IOWA
Great River Medical Center
West Burlington, IA

Mercy Medical Center, Cedar
Rapids
Cedar Rapids, IA

Mercy Medical Center, Sioux City
Sioux City, IA

St. Luke's Methodist Hospital
Cedar Rapids, IA

University of Iowa Hospitals and
Clinics
Iowa City, IA

KANSAS
Mercy Regional Health Center
Manhattan, KS

Shawnee Mission Medical Center
Merriam, KS

Shawnee Mission Medical Center
Shawnee Mission, KS

University of Kansas Hospital
Authority
Kansas City, KS

Via Christi Regional Medical
Center
Wichita, KS

KENTUCKY
Baptist Hospital East
Louisville, KY

Central Baptist Hospital
Lexington, KY

Jewish Hospital
Louisville, KY

St. Luke's Hospitals
Ft. Thomas, KY

University of Kentucky Hospital
Lexington, KY

University of Louisville Hospital
Louisville, KY

LOUISIANA
Christus St. Patrick Hospital
Lake Charles, LA

Kenner Regional Medical Center
Kenner, LA

Lindy Boggs Medical Center
New Orleans, LA

Louisiana Heart Hospital
Lacombe, LA

Ochsner Clinic Foundation
New Orleans, LA

Our Lady of Lourdes Regional
Medical Center
Lafayette, LA

West Jefferson Medical Center
Marrero, LA

MAINE
Maine Medical Center
Portland, ME

York Hospital[†]
Member, Massachusetts General
Hospital TeleStroke Network
York, ME

MARYLAND
Anne Arundel Medical Center
Annapolis, MD

Franklin Square Hospital Center
Baltimore, MD

Good Samaritan Hospital of
  Maryland
Baltimore, MD

Greater Baltimore Medical Center
Baltimore, MD

Harbor Hospital
Baltimore, MD

Johns Hopkins Bayview Medical
  Center
Baltimore, MD

Montgomery General Hospital
Olney, MD

National Institute of Neurological
  Disorders and Stroke (NINDS)
Bethesda, MD

Peninsula Regional Medical
  Center
Salisbury, MD

St. Agnes Hospital
Baltimore, MD

St. Joseph Medical Center
Towson, MD

St. Mary's Hospital*
Affiliated with University of
  Maryland's TeleStroke
  Network
Leonardtown, MD

Sinai Hospital of Baltimore
Baltimore, MD

Suburban Hospital
Bethesda, MD

Union Memorial Hospital
Baltimore, MD

University of Maryland Medical
  Center*
Brain Attack Team provides
  outreach program for rural
  Maryland
Baltimore, MD

MASSACHUSETTS
Addison Gilbert Hospital
Gloucester, MA

Anna Jaques Hospital
Newburyport, MA

Athol Memorial Hospital
Athol, MA

Bay State Medical Center
Springfield, MA

Berkshire Medical Center
Pittsfield, MA

Beverly Hospital
Beverly, MA

Beth Israel Deaconess Medical
  Center–Boston (West Campus)
Boston, MA

Beth Israel Deaconess Medical
  Center–Needham
Needham, MA

Boston Medical Center Menino
  Campus
Boston, MA

Brigham & Women's Hospital*
Provider, TeleStroke Network
Boston, MA

Brockton Hospital
Brockton, MA

Cambridge Health
  Alliance/Cambridge[†]
Cambridge, MA

Cambridge Health
  Alliance/Somerville
Somerville, MA

Cambridge Health
  Alliance/Whidden
Everett, MA

Cape Cod Hospital
Hyannis, MA

Caritas Carney Hospital
Boston, MA

Caritas Good Samaritan
Brockton, MA

Caritas Holy Family Hospital
Methuen, MA

Caritas Norwood Hospital
Norwood, MA

Caritas St. Elizabeth's Medical
   Center
Boston, MA

Charlton Memorial Hospital[†]
Fall River, MA

Clinton Hospital
Clinton, MA

Cooley Dickinson Hospital
Northampton, MA

Emerson Hospital
Concord, MA

Fairview Hospital
Great Barrington, MA

Falmouth Hospital[†]
Falmouth, MA

Faulkner Hospital
Boston, MA

Franklin Medical Center[†]
Greenfield, MA

Hallmark Health System Lawrence
   Memorial
Medford, MA

Hallmark Health System
   Melrose/Wakefield
Melrose, MA

Harrington Memorial Hospital[†]
Southbridge, MA

Health Alliance Hospital
Leominster, MA

Heywood Hospital
Gardner, MA

Holyoke Medical Center
Holyoke, MA

Jordan Hospital[†]
Plymouth, MA

Lahey Clinic—Mary and Arthur
   Clapham Hospital
Burlington, MA

Lawrence General Hospital
Lawrence, MA

Lowell General Hospital
Lowell, MA

Marlborough Hospital
Marlborough, MA

Martha's Vineyard Hospital[†]
Oak Bluffs, MA

Mary Lane Hospital
Ware, MA

Massachusetts General Hospital*
Provider, TeleStroke Network
Boston, MA

Mercy Hospital
Springfield, MA

Merrimack Valley Hospital
Haverhill, MA

MetroWest Medical Center—
   Framingham Campus
Framingham, MA

MetroWest Medical Center—
   Natick Campus
Natick, MA

Milford Regional Medical Center
Milford, MA

Milton Hospital[†]
Milton, MA

Morton Hospital
Taunton, MA

Mt. Auburn Hospital
Cambridge, MA

Nantucket Cottage Hospital[†]
Nantucket, MA

Nashoba Valley Medical Center[†]
Ayer, MA

Newton-Wellesley Hospital
Newton, MA

Noble Hospital
Westfield, MA

North Adams Regional Hospital
North Adams, MA

North Shore Medical Center—
Salem Hospital
Salem, MA

North Shore Medical Center—
Union Hospital
Lynn, MA

Quincy Medical Center
Quincy, MA

St. Anne's Hospital
Fall River, MA

St. Luke's Hospital[†]
New Bedford, MA

St. Vincent Hospital
Worcester, MA

Saints Memorial Medical Center
Lowell, MA

Somerville Hospital[†]
Somerville, MA

South Shore Hospital
South Weymouth, MA

Southcoast Hospitals
Group/Charlton
Fall River, MA

Southcoast Hospitals Group/St.
Luke's
New Bedford, MA

Southcoast Hospitals Group/Tobey
Wareham, MA

Sturdy Memorial Hospital
Attleboro, MA

Tobey Hospital[†]
Wareham, MA

Tufts–New England Medical
Center
Boston, MA

University of Massachusetts
Memorial Medical Center
Worcester, MA

Whidden Memorial Hospital[†]
Everett, MA

Winchester Hospital
Winchester, MA

Wing Memorial Hospital
Palmer, MA

MICHIGAN

Bixby Medical Center
Adrian, MI

Borgess Medical Center
Kalamazoo, MI

Bronson Methodist Hospital
Kalamazoo, MI

Detroit Receiving Hospital—
University Health Center
Detroit, MI

Field Neuroscience Institute
Saginaw, MI

Henry Ford Hospital
Detroit, MI

Herrick Memorial Hospital
Tecumseh, MI

Metropolitan Hospital
Grand Rapids, MI

Munson Medical Center
Traverse City, MI

Northern Michigan Hospital
Petoskey, MI

Providence Hospital and Medical
    Centers
Southfield, MI

St. Joseph Mercy Oakland
Pontiac, MI

St. Mary's Health Care
Grand Rapids, MI

St. Mary's of Michigan Medical
    Center
Saginaw, MI

Sparrow Hospital
Lansing, MI

Spectrum Health
Blodgett Campus and Butterworth
    Campus
Grand Rapids, MI

University of Michigan Health
    System
Ann Arbor, MI

Wayne State University Medical
    Center*
Provider, TeleStroke Network
Detroit, MI

William Beaumont Hospital
Royal Oak, MI

MINNESOTA
Abbott Northwestern Hospital
Minneapolis, MN

Fairview Southdale Hospital
South Edina, MN

North Memorial Medical Center
North Robbinsdale, MN

Park Nicollet Health Services
St. Louis Park, MN

Rice Memorial Hospital
Willmar, MN

St. John's Hospital
Maplewood, MN

St. Joseph's Hospital
Saint Paul, MN

United Hospital
Saint Paul, MN

Woodwinds Health Campus
Woodbury, MN

MISSISSIPPI
Memorial Hospital at Gulfport
Gulfport, MS

MISSOURI
Barnes-Jewish Hospital
St. Louis, MO

Cox Health Systems
Springfield, MO

Lee's Summit Hospital
Lee's Summit, MO

Lester E. Cox Medical Center
Springfield, MO

Mid-America Brain and Stroke
    Institute
Kansas City, MO

Moberly Regional Medical Center
Moberly, MO

Northeast Regional Medical
    Center
Kirksville, MO

Research Medical Center
Kansas City, MO

St. Anthony's Medical Center
Saint Louis, MO

St. Francis Medical Center
Cape Girardeau, MO

St. John's Regional Health Center
Springfield, MO

St. Louis University Hospital
St. Louis, MO

St. Luke's Hospital of Kansas City
Kansas City, MO

Southeast Missouri Hospital
Cape Girardeau, MO

MONTANA
Benefis Healthcare
Great Falls, MT

Billings Clinic
Billings, MT

Deaconess Billings Clinic
Billings, MT

St. Patrick's Hospital Center
Missoula, MT

St. Vincent Healthcare
Billings, MT

NEBRASKA
Bryan LGH Medical Center
Lincoln, NE

Creighton University Medical
   Center
Omaha, NE

Nebraska Heart Hospital
Lincoln, NE

Nebraska Medical Center
Omaha, NE

NEVADA
Renown Regional Medical Center
Reno, NV

St. Mary's Regional Medical
   Center
Reno, NV

Sunrise Hospital and Medical
   Center
Las Vegas, NV

Washoe Medical Center/Renown
   Regional
Reno, NV

NEW HAMPSHIRE
Elliot Hospital[†]
Member, Massachusetts
   General Hospital TeleStroke
   Network
Manchester, NH

NEW JERSEY
Atlanticare
Egg Harbor Township, NJ

Capital Health System
Trenton, NJ

Deborah Heart and Lung Center
Browns Mills, NJ

Englewood Hospital
Englewood, NJ

Hackensack University Medical
   Center
Hackensack, NJ

Holy Name Hospital
Teaneck, NJ

Jersey Shore University Medical
   Center
Neptune, NJ

Morristown Memorial Hospital
Morristown, NJ

Overlook Hospital
Summit, NJ

Riverview Medical Center
Red Bank, NJ

Robert Wood Johnson University
   Hospital
Hamilton, NJ

Robert Wood Johnson University
   Hospital
New Brunswick, NJ

St. Francis Medical Center
Trenton, NJ

St. Joseph's Regional Medical
  Center
Paterson, NJ

Shore Memorial Hospital
Somers Point, NJ

Underwood Memorial Hospital
Woodbury, NJ

Valley Health Systems
Ridgewood, NJ

Virtua Memorial Hospital
  Burlington County
Mt. Holly, NJ

NEW YORK

Albany Medical Center
Albany, NY

Albany Memorial Hospital
Albany, NY

Arnot Ogden Medical Center
Elmira, NY

Bellevue Hospital
New York, NY

Benedictine Hospital
Kingston, NY

Beth Israel Medical Center
Kings Highway Division
Brooklyn, NY

Beth Israel Medical Center
New York, NY

Bronx Lebanon Hospital Center
Concourse Division
Bronx, NY

Brookdale University Hospital
Brooklyn, NY

Brookhaven Memorial Hospital
  Medical Center
Patchogue, NY

Cabrini Medical Center
New York, NY

Cayuga Medical Center
Tompkins, NY

City Hospital Center
Elmhurst, NY

Columbia Presbyterian Medical
  Center
New York, NY

Coney Island Hospital
Brooklyn, NY

Corning Hospital
Corning, NY

Crouse Hospital
Syracuse, NY

Ellis Hospital
Schenectady, NY

Elmhurst Hospital Center
Elmhurst, NY

Faxton St. Luke's Health Care
  System
Oneida, NY

Flushing Hospital
Flushing, NY

Franklin Hospital Medical Center
Valley Stream, NY

Geneva General Hospital
Geneva, NY

Glen Cove Hospital
Glen Cove, NY

Good Samaritan Hospital Medical
  Center
Suffern, NY

Good Samaritan Hospital Medical
  Center
West Islip, NY

Harlem Hospital Center
New York, NY

Highland Hospital
Rochester, NY

Hudson Neurology and
    Neurophysiology
Sleepy Hollow, NY

Hudson Valley Hospital Center
Cortlandt Manor, NY

Jacobi Medical Center
Bronx, NY

Jamaica Hospital
Jamaica, NY

Kaleida Health
Buffalo, NY

Kings County Hospital
Brooklyn, NY

Kingston Hospital
Kingston, NY

Lenox Hill Hospital
New York, NY

Lincoln Medical and Mental
    Health Center
Bronx, NY

Long Beach Medical Center
Long Beach, NY

Long Island College Hospital
Brooklyn, NY

Long Island Jewish Hospital
New Hyde Park, NY

Long Island Jewish Medical
    Center
Queens, NY

Lutheran Medical Center
Brooklyn, NY

Maimonides Medical Center
Brooklyn, NY

Mary Immaculate Hospital
Queens, NY

Mary Imogene Bassett Hospital
Cooperstown, NY

Mather Memorial Hospital
Port Jefferson, NY

Mercy Medical Center
Bronx, NY

Metropolitan Hospital Center
New York, NY

Millard Fillmore Hospital, Gates
Buffalo, NY

Mohawk Valley Heart Institute
Utica, NY

Montefiore Medical Center
Moses Division
Bronx, NY

Mount Sinai Hospital
New York, NY

Mount Sinai Queens
Queens, NY

Mount Vernon Hospital
Mount Vernon, NY

New York Community Hospital
Brooklyn, NY

New York Hospital Medical Center
Queens, NY

New York Methodist
Brooklyn, NY

New York Presbyterian Hospital
Columbia Medical Center
New York, NY

New York Presbyterian Hospital
Weill Cornell Medical Center
New York, NY

New York Westchester Square
    Medical Center
Bronx, NY

North Shore Forest Hills Hospital
Forest Hills, NY

North Shore University Hospital
Glen Cove, NY

North Shore University Hospital
Plainview, NY

North Shore University Hospital
Syosset, NY

Northern Westchester Hospital
Mount Kisco, NY

Nyack Hospital
Nyack, NY

NYU Medical Center
New York, NY

Orange Regional Medical Center
Middletown, NY

Our Lady of Lourdes Memorial
   Hospital
Binghamton, NY

Parkway Hospital
Forest Hills, NY

Peninsula Hospital
Far Rockaway, NY

Richmond University Medical
   Center
Staten Island, NY

Rochester General Hospital
Rochester, NY

St. Barnabas Hospital
Bronx, NY

St. Catherine of Siena Medical
   Center
Smithtown, NY

St. Charles Hospital
Port Jefferson, NY

St. Francis Hospital
Poughkeepsie, NY

St. John's Riverside Hospital
Yonkers, NY

St. Joseph's Hospital
Elmira, NY

St. Joseph's Hospital
Erie, NY

St. Luke's Cornwall Hospital
Newburgh, NY

St. Luke's Roosevelt Division
New York, NY

St. Peter's Hospital
Albany, NY

St. Vincent's Hospital
New York, NY

St. Vincent's Staten Island Hospital
Staten Island, NY

Samaritan Hospital
Troy, NY

Sound Shore Medical Center
Bronx, NY

South Nassau Communities
   Hospital
Oceanside, NY

Southampton Hospital
Southampton, NY

Southside Hospital
Bay Shore, NY

Staten Island University
   Hospital–North
Staten Island, NY

Stony Brook University Hospital
Stony Brook, NY

Strong Memorial Hospital
Rochester, NY

SUNY Downstate Medical
   Center
Brooklyn, NY

SUNY Upstate Medical University
Syracuse, NY

Vassar Brothers Medical Center
Poughkeepsie, NY

Victory Hospital
Brooklyn, NY

Westchester Medical Center
Valhalla, NY

White Plains Hospital Center
White Plains, NY

Winthrop University Hospital
Mineola, NY

Woodhull Medical Center
Brooklyn, NY

Wyckoff Hospital
Brooklyn, NY

NORTH CAROLINA

Carolinas Medical Center
Charlotte, NC

Central Carolina Hospital
Sanford, NC

Clinical Research of Winston-
Salem
Winston-Salem, NC

Duke University Hospital
Durham, NC

Forsyth Medical Center
Winston-Salem, NC

High Point Regional Health
System
High Point, NC

Mission Hospital
Asheville, NC

Moses Cone Health System
Greensboro, NC

North Carolina Baptist Hospital
Winston-Salem, NC

Novant Health/South Piedmont
Region/Presbyterian Hospital
Charlotte, NC

Pitt County Memorial Hospital
Greenville, NC

Presbyterian Hospital
Charlotte, NC

Presbyterian Hospital
Huntersville, NC

Presbyterian Hospital
Matthews, NC

Rowan Regional Medical
Center
Salisbury, NC

Thomasville Medical Center
Thomasville, NC

University of North Carolina
Hospitals
Chapel Hill, NC

WakeMed Health
Raleigh, NC

NORTH DAKOTA

There is no designated stroke
center in the state at this time,
but a plan is under way for the
development of a stroke center
at MeritCare Hospital, Fargo,
ND

OHIO

Akron General Medical Center
Akron, OH

Aultman Hospital
Canton, OH

Cleveland Clinic Foundation
Cleveland, OH

Fairview Hospital
Cleveland, OH

Genesis Healthcare System
Zanesville, OH

Humility of Mary Health Partners
(HMHP)—St. Elizabeth Health
Center
Youngstown, OH

Kettering Medical Center
Kettering, OH

Kettering Medical Center—
Sycamore
Miamisburg, OH

Lake Hospital System
Painesville, OH

Lakewood Hospital
Lakewood, OH

Marietta Memorial Hospital
Marietta, OH

Marymount Hospital
Cleveland, OH

Medical University of Ohio
Toledo, OH

MetroHealth Medical System
Cleveland, OH

Miami Valley Hospital
Dayton, OH

Middletown Regional Hospital
Middletown, OH

Mt. Carmel Medical Center West
Columbus, OH

Ohio State University Hospital
Columbus, OH

Riverside Methodist Hospital
Columbus, OH

St. Elizabeth Health Center
Youngstown, OH

St. Rita's Medical Center
Lima, OH

Summa Health System
Akron, OH

University of Cincinnati Medical
Center
Cincinnati, OH

University Hospital
Cincinnati, OH

University Hospitals of Cleveland
Cleveland, OH

University Medical Center of
Ohio
Toledo, OH

OKLAHOMA

INTEGRIS Southwest Medical
Center
Oklahoma City, OK

Oklahoma University Medical
Center
Oklahoma City, OK

OREGON

Adventist Medical Center
Portland, OR

Legacy Good Samaritan Hospital
and Medical Center
Corvallis, OR

Legacy Meridian Park Hospital
Tualatin, OR

Legacy Portland Hospital
Portland, OR

Providence Portland Medical
Center
Portland, OR

Providence St. Vincent Medical
Center
Portland, OR

Rogue Valley Medical Center
Medford, OR

Sacred Heart Medical Center
Eugene, OR

PENNSYLVANIA

Abington Memorial Hospital
Abington, PA

Albert Einstein Medical Center
Philadelphia, PA

Allegheny General Hospital
Pittsburgh, PA

Altoona Regional Health System
Altoona, PA

Central Montgomery Medical
    Center
Lansdale, PA

Conemaugh Memorial Medical
    Center
Johnstown, PA

Dubois Regional Medical Center
Dubois, PA

Easton Hospital
Easton, PA

Ephrata Community Hospital
Ephrata, PA

HealthSouth Mechanicsburg
Mechanicsburg, PA

HealthSouth Rehabilitation
    Hospital
York, PA

Holy Redeemer Health System
Meadowbrook, PA

Lancaster General Hospital
Lancaster, PA

Lehigh Valley Hospital
Allentown, PA

Lehigh Valley Hospital,
    Muhlenburg
Bethlehem, PA

MCP Hahnemann University
Philadelphia, PA

Mercy Hospital of Pittsburgh
Pittsburgh, PA

Milton S. Hershey Medical
    Center
Hershey, PA

Moses Taylor Hospital
Scranton, PA

Nazareth Hospital
Philadelphia, PA

Reading Hospital and Medical
    Center
West Reading, PA

Riddle Memorial Hospital
Media, PA

St. Mary Medical Center
Langhorne, PA

Thomas Jefferson University
    Hospitals
Philadelphia, PA

University of Pennsylvania
    Hospital
Philadelphia, PA

University of Pittsburgh
Pittsburgh, PA

UPMC Presbyterian Shadyside
Pittsburgh, PA

RHODE ISLAND

Miriam Hospital
Providence, RI

SOUTH CAROLINA

AnMed Health
Anderson, SC

Greenville Hospital System
Greenville, SC

Medical University of South
Carolina
Charleston, SC

Providence Heart Institute
Columbia, SC

Roper Hospital
Charleston, SC

Spartanburg Regional Healthcare
System
Spartanburg, SC

SOUTH DAKOTA

Avera McKennan Hospital and
University Health Center
Sioux Falls, SD

Sioux Valley Hospital USD
Medical Center
Sioux Falls, SD

TENNESSEE

Baptist Hospital
Nashville, TN

Fort Sanders Regional Hospital
Knoxville, TN

St. Thomas Hospital
Nashville, TN

Seton Corporation d/b/a Baptist
Hospital
Nashville, TN

Skyline Medical Center
Nashville, TN

University of Tennessee
Memorial Hospital
Knoxville, TN

Vanderbilt University Hospital and
Vanderbilt Clinic
Nashville, TN

Wellmont Bristol Regional Medical
Center
Bristol, TN

TEXAS

Baylor University Medical Center
Dallas, TX

Brackenridge Hospital
Austin, TX

Citizens Medical Center
Victoria, TX

Columbia Medical Center
Arlington, TX

Denton Regional Medical Center
Denton, TX

DeTar Healthcare System
Victoria, TX

Doctors Hospital of Dallas
Dallas, TX

East Texas Medical Center Tyler
Tyler, TX

Harris Methodist Hospital
Fort Worth, TX

Heart Hospital of Austin
Austin, TX

Hillcrest Baptist Medical Center
Waco, TX

Medical Center of McKinney
McKinney, TX

Medical Center of Plano
Plano, TX

Medical City Dallas Hospital
Dallas, TX

Memorial Hermann Hospital
Houston, TX

Memorial Hermann Southwest
Hospital
Houston, TX

Memorial Hermann, The
Woodlands Hospital
The Woodlands, TX

Methodist Hospital
Houston, TX

Midland Memorial Hospital
Midland, TX

North Austin Medical Center
Austin, TX

Presbyterian Hospital of Dallas
Dallas, TX

Providence Memorial Hospital
El Paso, TX

Richardson Regional Medical
    Center
Richardson, TX

St. David's Medical Center
Austin, TX

St. Luke's Episcopal Hospital
Houston, TX

Scott and White Hospital and
    Clinic
Temple, TX

Seton Medical Center
Austin, TX

Sid Peterson Memorial Hospital
Kerrville, TX

Sierra Medical Center
El Paso, TX

Southwest Texas Methodist
    Hospital
San Antonio, TX

Tarrant County Hospital
Fort Worth, TX

United Regional Health Care
    System
Wichita Falls, TX

University Medical Center
Lubbock, TX

University of Texas Southwestern
    Medical Center
Dallas, TX

Valley Baptist Medical Center
Harlingen, TX

West Houston Medical Center
West Houston, TX

Wilson N. Jones Medical Center
Sherman, TX

UTAH

LDS Hospital
Salt Lake City, UT

University of Utah Allen Memorial
    Hospital*
Provider, TeleStroke Network
Salt Lake City, UT

Utah Valley Regional Medical
    Center/Orem Community
    Hospital
Provo, UT

VIRGINIA

Bon Secours—St. Mary's Hospital
Richmond, VA

Chippenham Medical Center
Johnston—Willis Hospital
Richmond, VA

Danville Regional Medical Center
Danville, VA

Inova Alexandria Hospital
Alexandria, VA

Inova Fairfax Hospital
Falls Church, VA

Riverside Regional Medical Center
Newport News, VA

Sentara Hospitals Norfolk
Norfolk, VA

Sentara Virginia Beach General
    Hospital
Virginia Beach, VA

University of Virginia Health
   System
Charlottesville, VA

Virginia Commonwealth
   University (VCU) Medical
   Center
Richmond, VA

Winchester Medical Center, Valley
   Health
Winchester, VA

WASHINGTON

Harborview Medical Center
Seattle, WA

Northwest Hospital and Medical
   Center
Seattle, WA

Overlake Hospital Medical
   Center
Bellevue, WA

Providence Everett Medical Center
Everett, WA

Providence St. Peter's Medical
   Center
Olympia, WA

Sacred Heart Medical Center
Spokane, WA

Southwest Washington Medical
   Center
Vancouver, WA

Swedish Medical Center
Seattle, WA

Swedish Medical
   Center/Providence
Seattle, WA

Valley Medical Center
Renton, WA

Virginia Mason Medical Center
Seattle, WA

WISCONSIN

Aurora BayCare Medical
   Center
Green Bay, WI

Aurora St. Luke's Medical
   Center
Milwaukee, WI

Bellin Hospital
Green Bay, WI

Columbia St. Mary's Hospital
Milwaukee, WI

Froedtert Memorial Lutheran
   Hospital
Milwaukee, WI

Gundersen Lutheran Medical
   Center
LaCrosse, WI

Luther Midelfort
Eau Claire, WI

Oconomowoc Memorial
   Hospital
Oconomowoc, WI

St. Agnes Hsopital
Fond du Lac, WI

St. Francis Hospital
Milwaukee, WI

St. Mary's Hospital Ozaukee
Meqwon, WI

St. Vincent Hospital
Green Bay, WI

Theda Clark Medical Center
Neenah, WI

Waukesha Memorial Hospital
Waukesha, WI

WEST VIRGINIA

Charleston Area Medical
   Center
Charleston, WV

St. Mary's Medical Center
Huntington, WV

West Virginia University
  Hospitals
Morgantown, WV

University of Wyoming Medical
  Center
Wyoming LifeFlight transports
  patients to the hospital's Trauma
  Center from rural areas in Wyo-
  ming and surrounding states
Casper, WY

Hyperbaric Oxygen Therapy

Freestanding hyperbaric oxygen therapy (HBOT) centers now exist in many states, in cities large and small. The challenge is finding them, because an FDA ruling prevents HBOT facilities from advertising that they provide stroke or other "off-label" hyberbaric treatments. Because the following centers do not advertise that they treat stroke, it took weeks of searching the Internet just to find them and then to check them out, Web site by Web site. But the effort was well worth it: I found more than a hundred of these facilities, in thirty-seven of the fifty states. Although no HBOT for stroke is covered by insurance, some of these centers offer payments on a sliding scale, according to income, and many offer reduced-rate accommodations on the premises or in nearby hotels or motels.

I have included the name of a medical doctor (M.D.) or an osteopathic physician (D.O.) per center (often there are more than one) if this information was given on the center's Web site. Listings without these names will need follow-up. Remember, no reputable HBOT facility operates without the supervision of a physician. For safety reasons, I also am not in favor of the inflatable for-home-use hyperbaric units unless treatments are closely monitored by a physician.

Because of the growing acceptance of HBOT within the medical profession, I also recommend updating my list by going to the following Web sites that provide directories of HBOT centers around the country:

- International Hyperbaric Association (www.internationalhyper baricassociation.org) is a nonprofit group whose mission is to promote universal access of HBOT for every medical condition it helps, especially brain injury, with a goal of full reimbursement by government and private insurance companies. It sponsors the National Parent to Parent Network (MUMS) for children who need HBOT. Their Web site (www.netnet.net/mums/) has a state-by-state database of hyperbaric treatment centers (these also treat adults), plus information about mobile HBOT units that travel around the country.

- Undersea and Hyperbaric Medical Society (www.uhms.org) has a state-by-state chamber directory of six hundred hospitals and freestanding centers that provide HBOT. This organization, however, does not endorse the use of HBOT for treating strokes. Nevertheless, I found more than twenty listings for HBOT centers—including the most well-known and highly reputable— that do treat strokes. Avoid listings for hospitals or clinics attached to hospitals, because they rarely provide HBOT for strokes. Limit your search to facilities listed as "clinic" or "medical," and then make sure they treat strokes.

- The directory at www.healthgrades.com/local-doctors-directory/ byspecialty/undersea-hyperbaric-medicine lists, by state and by city, the names of medical doctors who specialize in hyperbaric medicine. Ratings are also available for a fee. Finding a physician rather than a facility is a good approach, although follow-up will be needed to determine whether the hyperbaric physician treats strokes.

- Typing "Hyperbaric Oxygen for Stroke" into a search engine will bring up thirty thousand pages of listings—one of the disadvantages of using the Web! Try an advanced search by typing in a city and/or state after this phrase, enclosing the entire phrase in double quotes.

- International Alternative Medicine, USA (www.international altmed.com) has a list of HBOT centers that also will need follow-up as to whether they treat strokes.

- Medicaid for HBOT (www.medicaidforhbot.com) is a group for families with children who receive hyperbaric oxygen treatment for traumatic brain injury, including strokes and other medical conditions. The Web site provides updates on their campaign to win Medicaid reimbursement for HBOT for children. Members also share information in their chat room, which you may find useful.

HBOT Providers

The following list of freestanding centers that provide hyperbaric oxygen therapy is not a recommendation or an advertisement of their services. I have included a Web site or an email address in the listing wherever it was available, but I have not included telephone numbers, as too often I found that they were out of date.

ALABAMA

Hyperbaric Center of Alabama
Woodie Fritz, M.D.
www.hbotalabama.com
Birmingham, AL

ALASKA

American Hyperbaric Center
Robert Thompson, M.D.
www.americanhyperbariccenter.com
Anchorage/Wasilla, AK

ARIZONA

HBOT of Arizona
Howard Reuben, M.D.
www.hbotfaz.org
Phoenix, AZ

NorthStar Hyperbarics
Carol Henricks, M.D.
www.northstarhbot.com
Tuscon, AZ

Scottsdale Hyperbarics
www.scottsdalehyperbaric.com
Scottsdale, AZ

ARKANSAS

Arkansas Hyperbaric Association
William J. Lagaly, D.O.
Hot Springs, AR

CALIFORNIA

Beverly Hills Center for Hyperbaric
    Medicine
Ralph Potkin, M.D.
www.hyperbaricrx.com
Beverly Hills, CA

Health Restoration Center
David A. Steenblock, D.O.
www.strokedoctor.com
Mission Viejo, CA

California Hyperbaric
    Therapy
Geoffrey H. Saft, D.O.
www.hyperbaric-oxygen-ca.com
Corte Madera, CA

Central/Northern California
    Hyperbaric Center
Frederick S. Cramer, M.D.
www.hboinfo.com
Rhonert Park, CA

Chico Hyperbaric Center
Kurt Johnson, M.D.
www.HBOToday.com
Chico, CA

Developmental Spectrums
    Hyperbarics
Lynne R. Mielke, M.D.
www.spectrumh.com
Pleasanton, CA

Hyperbaric Oxygen Clinic of
  Sacramento
John Cassidy, M.D.
hbodoc@yahoo.com
Sacramento, CA

Hyperbaric Oxygen Clinic of Santa
  Monica
Michael Uszier, M.D.
www.hbot.info

Hyperbaric Oxygen Physical
  Enrichment Center
Phyllis Preciado, M.D.
(Soldiers who suffered traumatic
  brain injuries in Iraq and
  Afghanistan are treated without
  charge.)
www.hopeformychild.com
Fresno, CA

Hyperbaric Recovery and
  Rejuvenation Centers
www.hyuperbaricrecoverycenter
  .com
Rhonert Park, CA

A Natural Balance Integrative
  Wellness Center
Gary E. Foresman, M.D.
www.anaturalbalance.com
Arroyo Grande, CA

Orange County Wound and
  Hyperbaric
Darryl Werner, M.D.
www.woundandhyperbaric.com
Santa Ana, CA

Rancho Mirage Hyperbarics
Dr. Chuck Shapard
www.ranchomiragehyperbarics
  .com
Rancho Mirage, CA

Rapid Recovery Hyperbarics
Donald Underwood, D.O., M.D.
www.hbot4u.com
San Bernadino, CA

Sacramento Hyperbaric Center
Kurt Johnson, M.D.
www.HBOToday.com
Charmichael, CA

San Diego Center for Hyperbaric
  Therapy
David Bortz, M.D.
www.SCD4bot.com
San Diego, CA

San Diego Hyperbaric Centers
Harvy Tuomi, M.D.
www.hboinfo.com
San Diego, CA

Whitaker Wellness Institute
Julian Whitaker, M.D.
Mark Filidei, M.D.
Donald L. Jolly-Gabriel, Ph.D.
www.whitakerwellness.com
Newport Beach, CA

COLORADO

Calliste Medical
Kelly Z. Sennholz, M.D.
www.callistomedical.com
Denver, CO

Rocky Mountain Health Center
Alexander Thermos, D.O.
www.RockyMountainHealthCenter
  .com
Lakewood, CO

CONNECTICUT

Breiner Whole Body Health
  Centre
Adam Briener, M.D.
www.wholebodydentistry.com
Trumbell, CT

DISTRICT OF COLUMBIA

Natural Integrated Health
  Association
Bruce Rind, M.D.
www.drrind.com
Washington, D.C.

FLORIDA

Bay Medical Hospital Center
www.baymedical.org
Panama City, FL

Central Florida Hyperbaric
   Oxygen
Tracy Rhodes, M.D.
www.centralfloridahyperbarics.com
Winter Park, FL

Hyperbaric Medicine, Inc.
Albert E. Zant. M.D.
hbot913@aol.com
Destin and Fort Walton, FL

Hyperbaric Services of the Palm
   Beaches
Norman P. Ellison, M.D.
Hbotxofpalmbeach.com
Delray Beach, FL

National Hyperbarics
Allan Spiegel, M.D.
www.florida-oxygen.com
Palm Harbor, FL

Ocean Hyperbaric Neurologic
   Center
(Founded by the late Richard
   Neubauer, M.D.)
www.oceanhob.com
Lauderdale-by-the-Sea, FL

Perlmutter Hyperbaric Center
David Perlmutter, M.D.
www.perlhealth.com
Naples, FL

Physical Medicine and
   Rehabilitation
Thomas R. Murray, M.D.
ckressel@msn.com
Jacksonville, FL.

South Florida Center for H.O.P.E.
Jack S. Olin, M.D.
www.sfcenterforhope.com
Deerfield Beach, FL

GEORGIA

Atlanta Hyperbaric and Wound
   Care Clinic
Decatur, GA

Hyperbaric Physicians of Georgia
A group of twelve medical doctors
www.hbomdga.com
Marietta, GA

International Alternative Medicine
Edward P. Parrish III, M.D.
alternativemedic@aol.com
Tucker, GA

ProHBO at Health Horizons
Ken Knott, M.D.
www.prohbo.com
Marietta, GA

HAWAII

Hyperbaric Medicine Center of
   Hawaii
Hyperbaricmedicinecenter.com
Honolulu, HI

IDAHO

Idaho Hyperbarics
Portneuf Medical Center for
   Physical Therapy
Michael Baker, M.D.
www.idahobyperbarics.com
Pocatello, ID

ILLINOIS

Arlington Heights Longevity
   Institute
Terril Haws, D.O.
Arlington, IL

Harch Hyperbarics
Paul Harch, M.D.
www.harchhyperbarics.com
Chicago, IL

Midwest Hyperbaric Institute
August Martinacci, M.D.
www.midwesthbot.com
Bolingbrook, IL

INDIANA

Medical Center of South Indiana
New Albany, IN

Northern Indiana Hyperbarics
www.northernindianahyperbarics
   .com
Mishawaka, IN

Turner Clinic of Natural
   Medicine
Lafayette, IN

LOUISIANA

Family Physician Center
Paul Harch, M.D.
www.harchhyperbarics.com
Marrero, LA

Greenbriar Hyperbaric Unit
Eduardo J. Hernandez, M.D.
gbnh@bellsouth.com
Slidell, LA

MAINE

Integrative Wellness
www.integrativewellness.com
Portland, ME

MARYLAND

Center for Holistic Medicine
Rockville, MD

GBMC Health Care
Daniel John, M.D.
www.gbmc.org
Baltimore, MD

MASSACHUSETTS

Hyperbaric Oxygen Treatment
   Centers
Grace Doherty, M.D.
Randolph, MA

MICHIGAN

Macomb/Clinton Center for
   Wound Care and Hyperbaric
   Medicine
Richard Utranachitt, M.D.
www.hyperbaricandwoundcare.com
Clinton Township, MI

Metro Hyperbaric and Wound
   Healing Center
www.michiganhyperbaric.com
St. Clair Shores, MI

Vital Age Management
Robert Grafton, M.D.
vitalage@yahoo.com
Rochester Hills, MI

MINNESOTA

Life Force Therapies
www.lifeforcetherapiesusa.com
Plymouth, MN

Northwest Hyperbaric Services
Minneapolis, MN

MISSISSIPPI

Delta Region Medical Center
Greenville, MS

MISSOURI

Hyperbaric Healing Institute
Ganesh Gupta, M.D.
www.HHI-KC.com
Kansas City, MO

McDonagh Medical Center
Charles J. Rudolph, D.O.
www.mcdonaghmed.com
Kansas City, MO

NEVADA

Desert Hyperbarics
John Thompson, D.O.
www.deserthyperbarics.com
Las Vegas, NV

Hyperbaric Oxygen Clinic of
    Nevada
Reno, NV

Nevada Clinic
F. Fuller Royal, M.D.
Nevadaclinic.com
Las Vegas, NV

Nevada Institute of Hyperbaric
    Medicine
Henderson, NV

Northern Nevada Hyperbaric
    Center
Jonathan Tay, M.D.
www.nevadahyperbarics.com
Reno, NV

NEW JERSEY

First Step Achievements—Valley
    Health
Jo Feingold, M.D.
Hawthorne, NJ

New Jersey Hyperbaric Oxygen
    Therapy
Julia Bramwell, M.D.
www.njhbot.com
Parsippany, NJ

NEW MEXICO

Hyperbaric Medical of New
    Mexico
Kenneth P. Stoller, M.D.
www.hbotnm.com
Santa Fe, NM

NEW YORK

Hyperbaric Medicine of New York
Ahmed Abou-Taleb, M.D.
Great Neck, NY

Valley Health and Hyperbarics
Jo Feingold, M.D.
www.valleyhyperbarics.com
Brewster, NY

Whole Life Practices
www.wholelifepractices.com
North Bellmore, NY

NORTH CAROLINA

Medicor HBO
Dr. Joseph Jemsek
www.medicorhbo.com
Huntersville, NC

OHIO

Cole Center for Healing
Theodore J. Cole, D.O., N.M.D.
www.cincinnatihyperbarics.com
Cincinnati, OH

Dayton Ear, Nose and Throat
    Surgeons
John H. Boyles, M.D.
www.daytonent.com
Dayton, OH

Get Well Center
Hoyung Chung, D.O.
www.getwellcenterohio.com
Mansfield, OH

Preventive Medicine Group
Derrick Lonsdale, M.D.
www.prevmedgroup.com
Westlake, OH

OKLAHOMA

Hyperbaric Institute of Oklahoma
Sandy Price, M.D.
www.hyperbaricinstitute.com
Oklahoma City, OK

Jenks Health Team Hyperbarics
Gerald Wootan, D.O.
www.jenkshealthteam.com
Jenks, OK

New Hope Health Center
www.newhopehealthclinic.com
Tulsa, OK

OREGON

Integrated Medicine Group
www.integratedmedicinegroup.com
Portland, OR

OxyBioTech, Inc.
www.oxybiotech.net
Hillsboro, OR

PENNSYLVANIA

Hyperbaric Oxygen Medical Center
Lewis J. Neureater, M.D.
www.hboxygen.freeyellow.com
Columbia, PA

Mercy Wellness Center
Philadelphia, PA

Pinnacle Health
Raymond F. Kostin, M.D.
Mechanicsburg, PA

Pittsburgh Hyperbarics Institute
Frank Morganti, D.C.
John Lees, M.D.
www.pittsburghhyperbaric.com
Bridgeville, PA

Robert M. Lombard Hyperbaric
    Oxygen
Columbia, PA

SOUTH CAROLINA

Charleston Hyperbaric Medicine
Charles V. Percy, M.D.
hyperbar@bellsouth.net
Charleston, SC

TENNESSEE

Erlanger Medical Center
James Creel, M.D.
www.erlanger.org
Chattanooga, TN

TEXAS

Doctors Clinic
Gerald Parker, D.O.
www.doctorsclinicamarillo.com
Amarillo, TX

Hyperbaric Technologies
Akhtar Hossain, M.D.
www.hypertec-02.com
Olney, TX

Johnson Medical Associates
Alfred Johnson, D.O.
www.johnsonmedicalassociates.com
Richardson, TX

Lufkin Hyperbaric Center
Calvin Cargill, M.D.
www.lufkinhbo.com
Lufkin, TX

San Antonio Hyperbarics
www.sanantoniohyperbarics.com
San Antonio, TX

South Coast Hyperbaric Medicine
www.southcoasthyperbarics.com
Webster, TX

UTAH

National Hyperbaric Rehabilitation
    Center
Peter Clemens, M.D.
tpearce@utahhealingchamber.com
Taylorsville, UT

Utah Hyperbaric Oxygen Center
Larry D. Stoddard, M.D.
Layton, UT

Wasatch Hyperbaric Center
www.utahhealingchamber.com
Salt Lake City, UT

VIRGINIA

Comprehensive Medical Center for
    Integrative Medicine
Manjit R. Bajwa, M.D.
drbajwa11@yahoo.com
Alexander, VA

Mount Rogers Clinic
Edwardo Castro, M.D.
www.mtrogersclinic.com
Troutdale, VA

WASHINGTON

Hyperbaric Healing Center
James B. Wagner, Medical Director
www.hhc.com
Port Orchard, WA

National Health Medical Center
John F. Ruhland, M.D.
Seattle, WA

Spokane Hyperbaric Center
www.khyperbarics.com
Spokane, WA

WISCONSIN

Wilntey Hyperbaric Center
Madison/Fitchburg, WI

Wisconsin Hyperbaric Oxygen
   Center
www.whbot.org
Waterloo, WI

Wisconsin Integrative Hyperbaric
   Center
www.wisconsinhyperbarics.com
Fitchburg, Green Bay, Lacrosse,
   Eau Claire, and Milwaukee, WI

Integrative Medicine

Many of the HBOT centers in the immediately preceding list also provide holistic medical treatments. Words such as "alternative," "total health," "comprehensive," or "wellness" in the names of these centers are good indications that treatments besides hyperbaric are available. In addition, here are some excellent directories on the Web for integrative medical practitioners:

- www.webmed.com/content/pages/25/113599.htm provides a list of treatment centers, listed alphabetically by state. Click on "Finding an Integrative Medical Center."

- The Holistic Internet Community (www.holistic.com) provides more than thirteen hundred listings of holistic medical doctors, with details about each one. You can search by state or by the kind of treatment you are looking for.

- Alternative Medical Services (www.alternativeservicesdirectory .com) lists holistic physicians who practice in all fifty states.

- www.diagnoseme.com/region-A is a city-by-city listing of licensed holistic doctors. Type in the appropriate letter after the hyphen.

- www.holisticnetwork.com/directory allows you to search by category of treatment, from acupuncture to yoga.

Stroke Organizations

American Academy of Neurology
www.aan.com

American Academy of Physical
  Medicine and Rehabilitation
www.aapmr.org

American Board of Preventive
  Medicine
www.abprevmed.org

American Congress of
  Rehabilitation Medicine
www.acrm.org

American Heart Association
  and American Stroke
  Association
www.strokeassociation.org

American Nurses Association
www.nursingworld.org

American Occupational Therapy
  Association
www.aota.org

American Physical Therapy
  Association
www.apta.org

American Speech-Language-
  Hearing Association
www.asha.org

Americans with Disabilities Act
  Information
www.nod.org

Brain Aneurysm Foundation
www.bafound.org

Brain Attack Coalition
www.stroke-site.org

Brain SPECT Imaging
www.amenclinics.com
www.brainmattersinc.com/stroke

CARF: The Rehabilitation
  Accreditation Commission
www.carf.org

Children's Hemiplegia and Stroke
  Association
www.hemi-kids.org

CIS Biotech, Inc.
Gold Dot: a blood assay to predict
  stroke
cisbiotech.com

Clinical Trials
www.clinicaltrials.gov

Clinical Trials: Stroke Trials
  Directory
www.strokecenter.org/trials

Consumer Information
  Center/Medicare Information
www.pueblo.gas.gov

Hazel K. Goddess Fund for Stroke
  Research in Women
www.thegoddessfund.org

Independent Living Research
  Utilization
www.liv.org

Joint Commission for the
  Accreditation of Healthcare
  Organizations
www.jointcommission.org/Certifica
  tionProgram/PrimaryStroke
  Centers/

National Aphasia Association
www.aphasia.org

National Institute on Disability and
  Rehabilitation Research
www.ed.gov/offices/osers/nidrr

National Institute of Neurological
  Disorders and Stroke
www.nih.gov

National Stroke Association
www.stroke.org

Pediatric Stroke Network
www.PediatricStrokeNetwork.com

Social Security Administration
www.ssa.gov

SuperSlow fitness program
www.superslow.com

Visiting Nurse Associations of
America
www.vnaa.org

Workers' Compensation
Information
(Consult your local office in the
state government pages of your
telephone directory)

Organizations for Caregivers

Caregivers Handbook
www.strokesafe.org/handbook
An excellent, printable, 42-page
guide

Family Caregiver Alliance
www.caregiver.org

Family Caregiving 101
www.familycaregiving101.org

National Alliance for Caregiving
www.caregiving.org

National Family Caregivers
Association
www.nfcares.org

National Organization for
Empowering Caregivers
www.nofec.org

National Stroke Association:
Hope: The Stroke Recovery
Guide
www.stroke.org
A comprehensive informational
booklet for families

National Stroke Association: Lotsa
Helping Hands
www.stroke.org/site/PageServer?pa
gename=Strokelinks

National Stroke Association:
Support Group Directory
www.nsa.networkats.com
Search for a local support group by
zip code

Rosalynn Carter Institute for
Human Development
www.rci.gsw.edu

Well Spouse Foundation
www.wellspouse.org

Bibliography

The books, abstracts, and articles in this section provide detailed information about the treatments mentioned in this book. They address concerns that both you and your doctor may need to discuss.

Medical Books, Abstracts, and Articles

Al-Waili NS, et al. Hyperbaric oxygen in the treatment of patients with cerebral stroke, brain trauma, and neurologic disease. *Adv Ther* 2005;22(6):6599–678. A joint study that includes Mount Vernon Hospital, Westchester Medical Center, and New York Medical College. "The results of HBO therapy in the treatment of patients with stroke . . . are promising and warrant further investigation."

Carmichael M. "Stronger, Faster, Smarter." *Newsweek*, March 26, 2007. The connection between exercise and brain neurogenesis.

Chen A. Effective acupuncture therapy for stroke and cerebro-vascular disease: Part II. *Am J of Acupuncture* 1993;21(3):205–219.

Dambinova SA, et al. Blood test detecting autoantibodies to NMDA neuroreceptors for evaluation of patients with transient ischemic attack and stroke. *Clin Chem* 2003;49:1753–1762. The Gold Dot blood test for predicting stroke.

Frey JL, et al. tPA by telephone: extending the benefits of a comprehensive stroke center. *Neurology* 2005;64:154–156.

Harch, PG, McCullogh, V. *The Oxygen Revolution: Hyperbaric Oxygen Therapy*. Long Island City, N.Y.: Hatherleigh Press, 2007.

Hopwood V, et al. The effect of acupuncture on the motor recovery of the upper limb after stroke. *Physiotherapy* 1997;83:614–619.

Maxfield WS. Hyperbaric oxygen therapy in modern medicine. Hyperbaric Symposium: Hyperbaric Oxygen for Neurological Conditions, San Jose, CA, August 27, 2005.

————. SPECT brain scan shows brain function and has documented clinical response to hyperbaric oxygen therapy. Fifth Hyperbaric Oxygenation and the Recoverable Brain International Symposium, Ft. Lauderdale, FL, July 18–22, 2006.

National Institutes of Health. Acupuncture. Consensus Development Statement. Washington, DC, November 3–5, 1997. "Positive clinical reports."

Neubauer RA, Maxfield WS. The polemics of hyperbaric medicine. *J of Physicians and Surgeons* 2005;10:116.

Rymer MM, et al. Expanded modes of tissue plasminogen activator delivery in a comprehensive stroke center increases regional acute stroke interventions. *Stroke.* 2003;34:725–728.

Toole JF. Stroke research and the 21st century. *Arch Neurol* 2000;57:55.

Toole JF, Jack CR. Food (and vitamins) for thought. *Neurology* 2002;58:1449–1451.

Workman WT. Hyperbaric oxygen therapy and combat casualty care: a viable potential. *Military Medicine* 1989;154.3:111. "Future direction dictates immediate scientific and medical support for the use of this powerful treatment modality."

Survivors' Stories

Houston, Polly. *Stroke: Recovery with Oxygen.* Flagstaff, Ariz.: Best Publishing, 2005. A stroke survivor goes through HBOT at Chico Hyperbaric Center. Good information about her personal experience and hyperbaric treatment in general.

Taylor, Jill Bolte, Ph.D. *My Stroke of Insight: A Brain Scientist's Personal Journey.* 2006. www.drjilltaylor.com. The author describes, emotionally as well as scientifically, surviving and recovering from a hemorrhagic stroke.

Timothy, Megan. *Let Me Die Laughing.* Idyllwild, Calif.: Crone House, 2006. An entertaining and insightful account of recovering from traumatic brain injury.

Index

NOTE: Page references in *italics* refer to photos.